Lesson 12: Riding the waves of emotion   107

Lesson 13: A mountain of courage within   115

Lesson 14: The stories our emotions tell   123

Lesson 15: Beyond life's inevitable challenges   129

Lesson 16: Noticing reactivity   137

Lesson 17: Your child's mind   145

Lesson 18: The science of positivity and optimism   153

Lesson 19: Meaning making   161

Lesson 20: Equanimity   169

Lesson 21: Gratitude   177

Lesson 22: Compassion   185

Lesson 23: Savouring and the beginner's mind   195

Lesson 24: Attunement   203

Lesson 25: Mindful communication   213

Lesson 26: Mindfulness for two—a PAUSE practice   223

Conclusion   230

Acknowledgments   231

Resources   232

Index   236

MINDFULNESS
FOR MUMS
& DADS

To my husband, our precious children and our family
– this book is dedicated to you all.

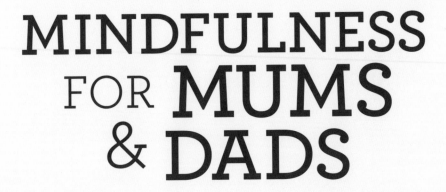

MINDFULNESS
FOR MUMS
& DADS

Proven strategies for calming down
and connecting

DR DIANA KOREVAAR

MURDOCH BOOKS
SYDNEY · LONDON

Contents

Introduction 7

Part One:
THE SCIENCE OF MINDFULNESS

Lesson 1: Wired for negativity 15

Lesson 2: A wandering mind is an unhappy mind 27

Lesson 3: Wired for connection 33

Lesson 4: Stress, strive or connect—
the three main circuits of emotion 41

Lesson 5: Connections and disconnections in families 49

Part Two:
PRACTICES AND TECHNIQUES TO TRY

Lesson 6: Meditation—a personal practice 59

Lesson 7: Meditation—body-based practices 65

Lesson 8: Meditation—breath practices 73

Lesson 9: Formal and informal practices 83

Lesson 10: Just this breath 91

Lesson 11: Inhabiting the body 99

Introduction

The world that we are living in and our children are growing up in is incredibly complex. It moves very quickly and the experience is often challenging. It is all too easy as a parent to get into an automatic pilot mode of living, simply pursuing one goal after another; in the process missing out on so much of the journey. In this book I hope to inspire you to step aside from the busy flow of life, and take advantage of the exciting developments in the field of neuroscience and mindfulness, by finding ways of applying the techniques to your own personal experience of life.

For most parents, attaining a sense of contentment and being at ease can all too often seem frustratingly elusive. What starts with the excitement (or pressure) of wanting to achieve a pregnancy, is often quickly replaced with worry—that check-ups will confirm things are 'normal' and that the child will be well. If, at the end of the pregnancy, we are presented with a healthy baby it can then feel as if a whole new world of things to worry about pours into our life. Why is this baby not sleeping? Is she getting enough milk? Why won't she stop crying? Am I doing the right things? And on it goes.

The trap we can easily fall into is coming to rely too heavily upon what is or isn't happening in order to feel okay. The experiences we get excited about—a new partner, a pregnancy or a holiday, at best provide only a temporary settling of this inner yearning for happiness.

Poet Rainer Maria Rilke writes of life:

> *Be patient toward all that is unsolved in your heart and try to love the questions themselves, like locked rooms and like books that are now written in a very foreign tongue. Do not now seek the answers, which cannot be given you because you would not be able to live them. And the point is, to live everything. Live the questions now. Perhaps you will then gradually, without noticing it, live along some distant day into the answer.*

If we dare to accept that these painful feelings of frustration, boredom or worry are not an indication that something is wrong, but are in fact integral to the experience of life and being a parent, then where does that actually leave us?

From my perspective as a perinatal psychiatrist, it leaves us in a more optimistic and exciting position than that of previous generations. Since the teaching of mindfulness was introduced to Western society over three decades ago, it has developed into a rich and diverse practice that lends itself perfectly to the task of enriching our relationships. Not only that, but when the techniques of mindfulness are incorporated in the way we parent our children, research suggests it is more likely they will develop greater emotional resilience, a quality that is more strongly associated with happiness in life than income or career.

However, the term 'mindfulness' has come to be used in many different ways and is used widely in a variety of settings, from the corporate world to education and even in the training of soldiers, which gets very confusing. Although mindfulness training programs in the area of psychology were initially designed to help manage stress, anxiety and depression, they evolved originally from more contemplative traditions such as Buddhism, where there was a much more direct process of inquiry into what it means to be human and live a meaningful life. There are now decades of accumulated research into the beneficial effects of mindfulness. It has been shown that regular practice leads to improvement in physical health as well as emotional wellbeing and also creates significant changes in the structure of our brains in a process which scientists have labelled neuroplasticity.

This term refers to the capacity of the brain to quite literally grow new nerve cell connections, based upon the patterns of our thinking and our behaviour. In other words, the more we 'practise' certain thinking patterns or behaviour the more strongly this circuitry gets reinforced within our nervous system, or in other words—'nerve cells that fire together, wire together'.

MRI scans of the brains of participants in mindfulness training courses such as Mindfulness Based Stress Reduction show that with only a few weeks of daily practice, there are measurable changes in brain structure. The small structure in the limbic system responsible for the secretion of the stress hormone cortisol reduces in size over the eight-week period, and areas in the frontal lobe of the brain responsible for balancing emotion, creative thinking, insight and wisdom increase in size.

Over recent years there have been two additional adaptations to traditional mindfulness training, which enable the skills to be of more practical use to parents. These two extra 'arms' of training focus more specifically upon emotion (balancing fear-based emotions with those of courage, kindness and self-compassion) and deepening connection in relationships, in a process which is called 'attunement'.

The last decade or so of research demonstrates how it is possible to shape underlying personality characteristics that were previously regarded as stable or fixed. For example, if genes and early life experiences have tended to make us self-critical, irritable or unable to read the emotions of others with accuracy, regular practice and use of mindfulness skills can bring about significant change.

However, when we are able to integrate mindfulness skills into daily life, we are not the only ones who benefit. Research shows how our emotions don't just shape the structure and activity of our own brains, but the brains of those around us! Mindfulness skills are now core components of training courses in parenting and in education settings because they help children grow into confident adults who are able to flourish in their social relationships, their emotional lives and in their capacity to learn and succeed in life more broadly.

Emeritus Professor Jon Kabat-Zinn is regarded by many as the father of Western mindfulness training. In his book *Wherever You Go, There You Are* he describes the way his own experience of becoming a parent deeply challenged and ultimately transformed his own practice of mindfulness. He came to regard the birth of each of his children as the arrival of a 'little Buddha or Zen master', effectively providing him with his own 'private mindfulness teacher'. The role of these little masters, he says, was to challenge every belief and limit he had, providing him with constant opportunities to recognise the things he was attached to, and to let them go. In this way he came to see parenthood as a long mindfulness retreat.

My own introduction to the experience of mindfulness began over fifteen years ago, when I found my way to a mindfulness teacher at a time when stress was taking a toll on my life. Unsure at the time of what was about to happen, my memory now is of meeting a rather physically imposing yet kind and softly spoken therapist, who allowed me to tell my story without interrupting, then led me through what I now recognise to have been a deep body scan. It was a powerful experience of feeling strong emotions. Fear, sadness and regret washed over me while awareness of body sensations seemed to provide a stable anchor for me.

I walked out of the therapist's consulting room feeling unexpectedly renewed. My body felt lighter, less tight and contracted, and the story I had told had shifted with regard to the meaning it held for me. Self-criticism and worry had subsided, and in their place were threads of kindness and a sense of optimism for the future.

I had learned a powerful lesson. As a result of that experience, but with no formal mindfulness training at that stage, I more intuitively understood the benefit of finding the courage to simply observe the feelings and stories I was bringing into my own experience of being a mother. From that time I engaged in various formal learning experiences, which were fundamentally quite different from my training as a doctor and psychiatrist, which had been based upon a more limited model of diagnosing and treating illness.

With the support of many inspiring teachers, over the last two decades I have steadily built my own nourishing practice of mindfulness. My children are all adults now, and thankfully for them, I believe, my training in mindfulness has allowed me to be more discerning in understanding their experiences of life and providing them with the support they need.

Working in the area of perinatal psychiatry, I see women and their families for many different reasons. Occasionally illness such as depression or anxiety needs to be managed, and then medication can play a useful role in improving not only mood and motivation, but also the capacity of the nervous system to access the concentration and focus required for creativity, new learning and potentially training in mindfulness.

As I became more confident with the techniques, I found that even when quite unwell, most patients valued learning about how stress affected the way their minds worked. As they experimented with mindfulness skills, they became more curious and less frightened of the activity of their minds, and their need for medication was often greatly reduced. Most of the patients I work with come to find the skills so essential and rewarding to use, that sooner or later they enrol in an eight-week formal mindfulness training program. Following that they rarely look back.

This book was inspired by a desire to interest more parents in the process of self-discovery that mindfulness training involves. I have tried to write this book in such a way that it is a lived experience, and as such in each chapter you will be invited to reflect upon your own emotional experience of life or of being in relationships. You will find instruction for formal meditation practice, but you will also read stories drawn from my own work with young parents (whose names have been changed in this book) who have found ways to integrate mindfulness into their lives.

Feel free to dip into chapters about subjects that catch your attention. There is no real need to read this book from beginning to end. In general, the early chapters provide background information about how our minds work and the source of mindfulness. The later chapters explore ways to bring mindfulness into our daily lives and relationships.

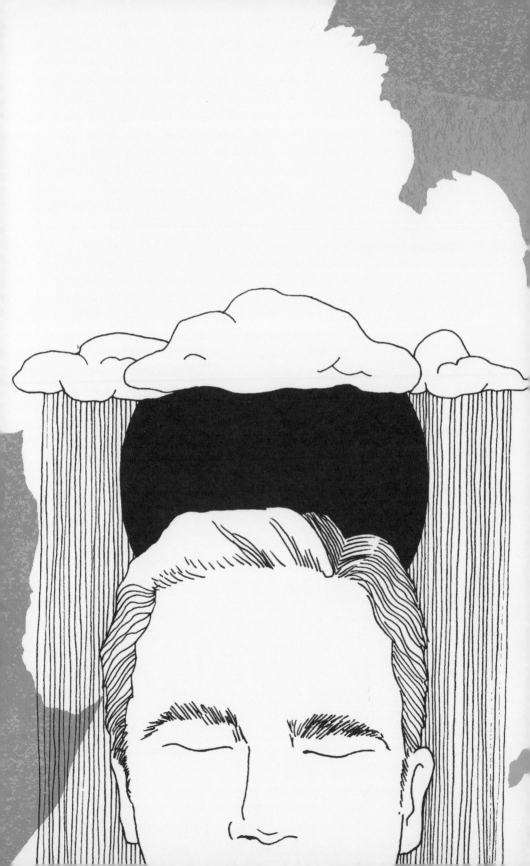

Part One

THE SCIENCE OF MINDFULNESS

Wired for negativity

The field of neuroscience has revealed a lot of information about how the human brain works, and why we are so vulnerable to stress. As humans, we have evolved over thousands of years, from species that survived only because they were good enough at protecting themselves from threat. But in Western society the threat is rarely located in our physical environment, so we live with the legacy of a powerful negative bias. The upshot is that the brains we are born with have many design features suited for a completely different era—when on a daily basis threats to life were routine.

In case you hadn't noticed, we have little control over our thoughts. Our genetic makeup and past experience play a big part in determining the thoughts we have and how we interpret experiences. In fact only 10 per cent of the activity of our brain is in conscious awareness, which is why attempting to simply change our thoughts is bound to fail. Whether they are optimistic thoughts or come in the form of worry or negativity is largely beyond our direct control. Our thoughts are intimately linked to emotion, which originates well beneath conscious awareness, in an area of the brain called the limbic system.

Scientific investigation into our vulnerability to stress has highlighted the role of a small structure located deep within the brain called the amygdala, which functions like a smoke detector—constantly vigilant for what might pose a threat or get in the way of an outcome we want. The big problem is that the amygdala has a hair-trigger. It can fire up when we feel frustrated by waiting in a long queue at the supermarket, or when we hear a particular tone in the voice of someone we are close to.

... the brains we are born with have many design features suited for a completely different era—when on a daily basis threats to life were routine.

When activity in the amygdala increases, the level of the stress hormone cortisol rises and blood is diverted away from areas in the brain that we rely upon for clear thinking and problem-solving.

We call this the 'stress response'. It may have helped our ancestors escape from predators, but it rarely helps us deal skilfully with challenges we face in day-to-day life.

For this reason, under the influence of negative emotions like anxiety, worry, irritability or anger, the functions of the frontal lobes of our brain are significantly impaired. These 'executive functions' give us the capacity to concentrate, make wise decisions and be creative. Being deprived of access to these skills contributes to processing problems, which in turn feeds the spiral of escalating negativity we become familiar with when we are stressed.

The strong bias in favour of detecting threat ensures that memories laid down most strongly (in the limbic system where the amygdala is located) are the negative ones. This means that we are more likely to remember a situation from years ago when we were criticised or blamed for something than we are to remember when we were praised. Neuropsychologist Rick Hanson describes our nervous system as being like 'Velcro' for negative events and 'Teflon' for good experiences.

Putting all this together, it is hardly surprising that pregnancy and childbirth is a time of increased risk of emotional disorders. Sleep deprivation and hormonal change generally tend to magnify the biological stress response, predisposing to illness that, even when it's mild, can impact greatly upon the experience of parenting.

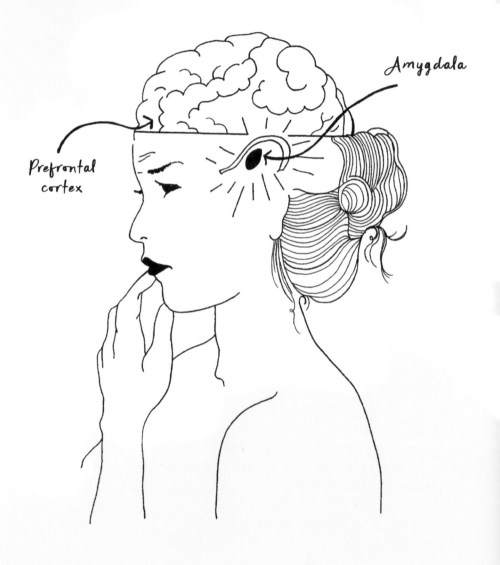

Amygdala

Prefrontal cortex

The amygdala is the part of the brain hardwired to detect threats

Although much of the focus tends to be on women and how they manage pregnancy and the postpartum months, we have to remember that from an emotional perspective new fathers are also at increased risk of becoming depressed and anxious. In fact, research suggests that depression is more likely to go unnoticed in men than in women, perhaps because they feel ashamed of not coping and are less confident talking about their feelings.

Jonathan's story

Jonathan and Katie's second child was three months old when Jonathan came to see me, concerned about his irritability and difficulty concentrating. Their young daughter Lyla had been born ten weeks prematurely and although she was doing very well, Jonathan felt that he was now really struggling to manage. He had returned to work six weeks after Lyla was born and he was still trying to help Katie with night feeds whenever he could.

For Jonathan, it felt as if life consisted only of work and worry. In the office it felt like a struggle to make the most basic of decisions, and at home his irritability was spilling out all over the place. Jonathan was finding himself getting angry with his three-year-old son Thomas and had begun to feel resentful of getting up in the middle of the night to tend to Lyla. He barely remembered what it was like to be able to rely on the friendship he had previously known with Katie for support. To Jonathan, it appeared as if his wife was totally consumed by the needs of their two young children and her own tiredness.

Katie was clearly distressed about her husband's irritability and, as we talked, it was clear that Jonathan was feeling deeply worried about the way his whole personality appeared to be changing.

As we explored more deeply what was going on for Jonathan it became apparent there were two different sorts of thought patterns happening. The first was a relatively straightforward process of worrying about the future, and the most significant example of this was his constant preoccupation with money. Jonathan had become particularly concerned about how he would be able to cope with doing the amount of work needed in order to earn enough money to pay the family's living expenses now that he was the only person generating an income for the family.

But there was also a different type of negativity going on for Jonathan, an even more painful experience for him to bear. Jonathan was beginning to believe that there was something fundamentally flawed about him, and I could feel his inner torment when he said, 'What sort of loser yells at their three-year-old son and gets annoyed with his wife who has just gone through the stressful experience of a premature birth.'

It is common for the early months of caring for a newborn to feel very isolating. Since Lyla was born, Jonathan had not managed to find time for either going to the gym or catching up with his friends. And the less Jonathan saw of his close friends, the more likely it would be that he would not get the reassurance he so badly needed—that he need not feel alone, that in fact the majority of young fathers go through periods of struggling with the experience of parenting.

What was complicating things further was the impact that stress was having on Jonathan's capacity to process information. He was getting a firsthand experience of how stress affects the way the brain works. If we had measured Jonathan's level of cortisol, the stress hormone, it would almost certainly have been higher than at other times when he was feeling at ease, and if we had done a brain scan I would expect that the size of his amygdala would be larger than normal, because he had experienced months of poor sleep, anxiety and low mood. Similarly, if we had specifically measured his memory function, concentration and capacity for lateral thinking and creativity they would almost certainly have been reduced.

In a practical sense, the impact that stress was having on how Jonathan's mind was processing information was likely to have been contributing significantly to his experience of depressed mood and irritability. Through no fault of his own, the negativity bias that was hardwired in Jonathan's brain was ensuring that more attention was being paid to what was not going well (Velcro brain) than more neutral or positive experiences (Teflon brain). He was so caught up in the busy activity of his mind that he was failing to pay attention to the warm hugs Thomas gave him or even notice Katie's smile as she watched him nursing Lyla.

But this story has an inspiring ending. Within a few months, Jonathan was feeling very different indeed. In our last session together he even said to me:

'I know this might sound crazy, but in a strange way I'm actually pleased that I hit a wall after Lyla was born. I was running on automatic pilot in my life, things had been going well but I was taking it all for granted and I came unstuck in a big way. I can see now that when things started to get hard, the first thing I did was blame myself for not trying harder. Now that I'm feeling different I can see just how easy it is to simply push harder. That is the only way I've ever known. I don't like the sort of person I became in those months after Lyla was born, but I think what I've learned about myself is going to change the sort of father I will be and the way I am in my relationship with Katie. I know when I first came here you were so worried that you thought I should consider taking medication. I'm glad now that I refused. Learning mindfulness has really changed me, and changed the way I am in my family.'

In Lesson 6 we meet Jonathan again when we look more closely at the specific mindfulness practices that form part of the mindfulness training techniques.

Very occasionally, postnatal illness in women can be much more severe.

Let's look now at just such a situation, where illness following childbirth led to a major breakdown in information processing within the brain.

Julie's story

Julie was referred to me a week after the birth of her first baby. Up until the 36th week of pregnancy she had worked as a chief executive officer in a multinational corporation. Although she was not unfamiliar with stress, it had never got in the way of her capacity to work and lead a full life.

Following a completely normal pregnancy and delivery, Julie developed postnatal psychosis. During a psychotic illness, connection with reality is lost, in an often terrifying way. Those affected occasionally hear inner voices as if they were real, misinterpret what is happening around them and become suspicious of seemingly normal events for reasons which are rarely clear to others.

Typical of such postnatal illness, Julie's symptoms fluctuated wildly. When she was more settled she was able to speak quite coherently about past life experiences, her pregnancy and her marriage. But when psychotic symptoms took over, things dramatically changed. Julie appeared terrified; she started shouting, crying and trying to communicate, but even for me as her psychiatrist, it was difficult to make sense of what her inner experience might be about.

Antipsychotic medication was crucial and it helped settle Julie's mental state and allowed her to get some sleep. Within 48 hours the intensity of her psychotic symptoms had reduced to the extent that we could discuss what was actually going on. With her husband present I explained to them both how the processing of even simple information within Julie's brain was very impaired as a result of sleep deprivation and hormonal change. As they battled to make sense of what was happening, a logical explanation of the anatomy of the stress response helped give them hope for the future.

Despite Julia's illness, her intermittent capacity to pay attention to our conversations suggested to me that she might be capable of using mindfulness exercises to build her ability to concentrate and focus her attention. As unwell as she was, Julie was relieved to find there was a way in which she could actively participate in her recovery, and she became an enthusiastic student of mindfulness. Ward nurses found a CD player, and when her thoughts were more organised and logical she began to follow instructions for a body scan meditation.

The practices transformed her. She explained later that they gave her a reassuring sense that she could work with her own mind and not be so frightened by thoughts, images and sounds which intermittently took over. Although she found the practice challenging, concentrating upon sensations in her body helped her feel as if she was getting some distance from the chaos of her mind.

When her baby was brought to her, Julie was able to hold him and use slow, stable breathing to build her capacity to concentrate. Over the next week she became slowly more confident in holding the focus of her attention in such a way that she could connect to the present moment, feeling the small body of her young son in her arms.

Over the following weeks and months, as we worked together to consolidate her recovery and make sense of what might have contributed to her severe illness, it became clear that as with many serious emotional disorders, Julie's postnatal psychosis was probably linked to traumatic experiences she had as a young child. Within Julie's brain, 'trauma circuits' had been reactivated after the birth of her son. During her experience of psychosis it was as if she'd been taken right back to childhood, reliving experiences she'd had years previously.

It was crucial to Julie's recovery that she made sense of what had happened but, as you can imagine, the process of therapy was at times quite tough. During her weekly sessions with me, we also worked on building Julie's confidence with mindfulness. She came to see that daily yoga stretches and body scans helped ground her in the present moment, allowing her to get some distance from what was coming up in therapy. But the practices also gave her a way of caring for herself and building a sense of inner strength, which was very different from simply distracting herself.

Most of us barely notice how frequently we use distraction as a way of avoiding uncomfortable feelings, thoughts or situations. However, rather than encouraging a settling of the mind, distraction tends to work by adding more 'white noise'. In the short term we might find this helpful, but more often distraction simply doesn't provide the respite we are looking for. During her pregnancy, when Julie was frantically juggling the demands of her busy home and work life, worry about how she might cope with being a mother began to emerge. Months later, after recovering from her illness, Julie came to understand just how frequently she used activities like surfing the internet, eating and even listening to music as ways of diverting her attention from worried thoughts or uncomfortable emotions.

Most of us barely notice how frequently we use distraction as a way of avoiding uncomfortable feelings, thoughts or situations.

As the months passed and Julie gained confidence with her mindfulness practice, she found it particularly helpful to target times when she felt an urge to distract herself, as an opportunity for observing more closely what was really going on in her mind.

Reflection

Just like any other organ in the body, there are many reasons why the function of the human brain might be temporarily impaired. Its capacity to process and recall information, think creatively and manage strong emotion can all be profoundly compromised by experiences as simple as sleep deprivation. Have you ever noticed that you handle challenging situations differently when you are tired? Is there a typical way that you feel about yourself or your life when you're tired which differs from how you feel when you are well rested and energised? ■

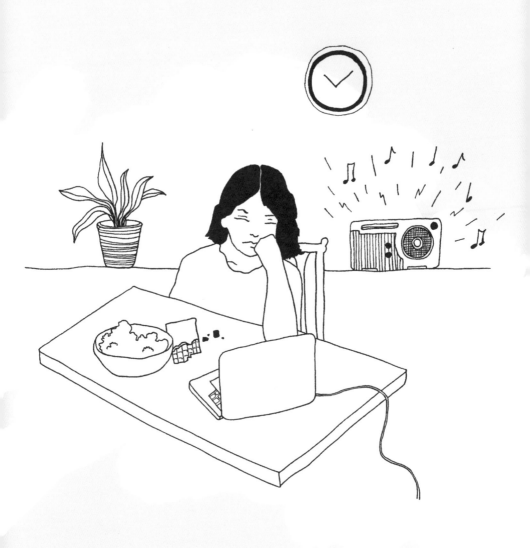

Multi-tasking can drain us of energy and create disconnection

A wandering mind is an unhappy mind

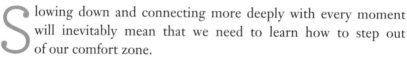

Slowing down and connecting more deeply with every moment will inevitably mean that we need to learn how to step out of our comfort zone.

A happy life—it's what we all hope for and want for those we care about. Yet even though we might strive to achieve goals and have precious possessions, research tells us that a happy life is more about our ability to be deeply engaged in the life we have. It is now believed that happiness and wellbeing are skills which are learned, much like riding a bicycle or playing a musical instrument.

How can this possibly be, you may ask, when life involves a lot of hard work, and at least some of the time, there may not seem to be much to show for it. Even when we are not facing any major challenges, juggling the demands of everyday life can feel like a treadmill of mundane and meaningless tasks. And if this is not enough, the decisions we make for our children are often influenced by the inevitable negative bias that filters into our lives through newspapers and television—graphic images of crime and human tragedy. It is hardly surprising that safety and security become our somewhat hidden priorities.

One of the most rewarding aspects of my job as a psychiatrist is working with parents and getting the opportunity to observe how challenges in life have the capacity to bring out strength, courage and wisdom in those who had initially turned to me at times when they felt lost and afraid. As hard as it may feel at the time, the only opportunities we really get to build inner strength and wisdom are when we are facing life's challenges.

But for this important growth to occur, it is essential that we are able to look with curiosity and without judgement at the areas of our life which are causing us pain. When we pay careful attention to what is feeling uncomfortable, we are able to find *the edge* at which growth can occur.

One of the characteristics of how the human mind works which makes it so vulnerable to stress and worry is its inherent tendency for mind wandering and multi-tasking. When our minds wander we are effectively disconnected from rich detail around us in the present moment. At those times we live in a 'virtual world', and it's *Mind wandering is generally the cause and not just the consequence of unhappiness.* not a happy world. The negativity bias which is hardwired as a result of the evolutionary priority to detect threat and prioritise survival, influences what we take notice of, what we ignore, and what does not even reach conscious awareness.

In a research project reported in the journal *Science* in 2010 titled 'A Wandering Mind Is an Unhappy Mind', scientists from Harvard University used a mobile phone app to check in on over 2,000 participants at random times during the day. They rated how often people's minds were wandering, what topics they wandered to and how it affected their mood. The research showed that people were experiencing mind wandering for almost 50 per cent of the time. Results of the research suggested that people were happiest when making love, exercising or engaging in conversation. They were least happy when resting, working or using a home computer. The researchers found that even when minds wander to pleasant topics they were no happier than when they were more fully engaged in their current activity. So while scientists had previously known that negative moods are more likely to be associated with mind wandering, this research provided evidence that mind wandering was generally the cause and not just the consequence of unhappiness.

It's impossible to stop thinking, but with training we become much better at recognising when we are caught up in repetitive cycles of worry and negativity.

Most of what drives our behaviour results from activity going on in our brains beneath conscious awareness. This is why many people struggle with overeating or using medication or alcohol in order to relax, trying usually in vain to get relief from the inner turmoil generated by untrained minds. In a similar way to what happens when we use physical exercise to build strength in our muscles, mindfulness training strengthens our capacity to concentrate, pay attention and direct the focus of our awareness in ways that we choose.

Mindfulness training is often misunderstood as a process of stopping thoughts or controlling emotion. It's impossible to stop thinking, but with training we become much better at recognising when we are caught up in repetitive cycles of worry and negativity.

We are beginning to understand how mindfulness has its effect upon the way the brain works, and why it has such a significant impact upon the actual structure of the brain. Research shows that an initial intense wave of negative emotion such as fear or anger, rising up from beneath conscious awareness, happens in all of us in much the same way. However, in those with mindfulness skills, negative emotion appears to be recognised much earlier, bringing with it an opportunity to pay more discerning attention to what is going on, which in turn reduces the opportunity for what we call rumination—the tendency to get caught up in loops of negative thinking. Compared with those who live life on 'automatic pilot', the trained mind appears to return to a state of emotional balance much more rapidly, allowing an opportunity for a more flexible response to what is happening.

Research also shows us that the more we practise particular emotions, the stronger they get, and the areas of the brain which produce these emotions become larger. The more we get caught up in worry, the better we get at it!

In mindfulness training we learn how to resist the tendency of our minds to wander by using anchors for our attention in the present moment. We might choose to 'connect' to the movement of our breath or sensations in our body, and whenever we do this we are re-educating our minds, and quite literally rewiring our brains. When we are with others and remember to ground our attention, we are able to tune in more carefully to what they might be trying to tell us, not only in their speech, but in the tone of their voice and in their behaviour.

As we will learn in subsequent chapters, building strength in the pathways connecting the process of breathing and body sensations to the brain helps create earlier recognition of anxiety, irritability and other emotions which are likely to influence our behaviour in unhelpful ways. Similarly, regularly grounding our attention and connecting more deeply to what is actually happening in the present moment makes it much more likely that we won't miss out on precious experiences which might otherwise pass by us unnoticed.

It is especially when we are with others that our capacity to be more grounded in the moment pays dividends. In the relationships we have with our partners and children, most of us notice how much more likely we are to be triggered into reacting with frustration or irritability when our minds are distracted or we are overly focused on getting tasks done.

Choosing to be mindful involves stepping out of what might feel like a comfort zone of distraction by turning again and again towards what is actually happening in the moment. In time our minds feel more robust and stable and we are less likely to react in impulsive ways. By coming to understand our own particular habits of reactivity we also develop a valuable capacity for insight, which in turn helps build a richer understanding of life experiences.

Reflection

How well does distraction work for you? What are the favourite activities you turn to for distraction, and do you move on from them feeling more or less relaxed, and more or less connected with life? ■

Lesson 3

Wired for connection

From the moment we are born we are hardwired to pick up on the emotions of those around us. Newborn babies shown simple images of a face will turn towards a drawing which shows a face with a smile and turn away from an image of a frowning face.

Mirror neurones—this is the name scientists have given to special nerve cells within the brain that appear to communicate information about emotion, and account for the fact that in our relationships we are quite literally influencing activity and ultimately the structure of each other's brains.

The 'still face experiment' is the name given to groundbreaking research back in the 1970s by Dr Ed Tronick, a developmental psychologist who demonstrated the capacity of even young babies to register and respond to the emotions of adults they interact with. In one video of the still face experiment (which can be seen on the internet) a mother and her twelve-month-old baby are initially observed engaging in a warm interaction. The young child is animated and smiling, pointing to things in the room, and the mother smiles too as she shares the experience, following the leads her baby gives her.

After a few minutes the mother turns her head to look away from the baby, and then as instructed by the researcher, she turns to face her baby again, but this time with a completely neutral and unreactive facial expression. We watch as the baby appears to try and get her mother to interact by looking closely at her, pointing and making noises. However, as the seconds pass and the baby is unable to get any response from her mother, she becomes unsettled. Initially she calls out and waves her arms, but when her mother continues to show no reaction at all, her distress quickly escalates.

Even though the baby is getting a neutral response from her mother's expression, she experiences negative emotion. As the seconds pass, it becomes clear that her inability to connect with her mother is activating a powerful reaction.

As the experiment proceeds to its conclusion, we watch mother and baby reconnect as the mother once again tunes in to the messages her baby is giving her, using a soothing voice and gentle touch to reassure her baby. *Babies shown simple images of a face will turn towards a drawing which shows a face with a smile and turn away from an image of a frowning face.* The bond between them is restored, and we see how rapidly the baby responds. Once again she is calm and settled.

This simple experiment demonstrated just how influential the emotional connections we have with each other are, and the findings continue to shape not only the course of child psychology and approaches to parenting, but also interventions in family and couple therapy.

As parents we are all familiar with how the busyness and demands of life can lead to a focus not on connecting, but on outcomes—'Is that homework done yet?'; 'Will we get a tantrum at swimming today?'; 'She better show some respect to her grandmother this evening!' On automatic pilot, looking for outcomes in relationships, we are not taking into consideration how emotions and behaviour impact directly upon how our brains work. In the still face experiment, different nerve cell circuitry is being activated depending upon whether the emotions of mother and child are tuned in to each other or not.

The human brain is an incredibly complex organ. It is a bit like a three-dimensional circuit board of nerve cells bathed in fluid in which

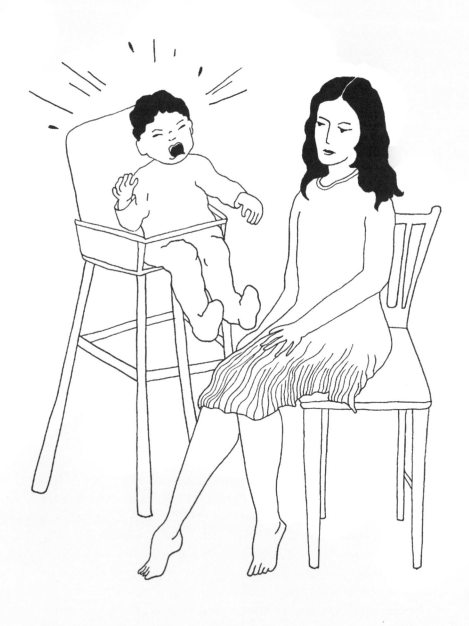

Babies respond to the emotions of the adults they interact with

chemicals (neurotransmitters) and hormones are suspended. Our brains consist of roughly ten billion nerve cells, with each cell forming complex connections to approximately 10,000 neighbouring cells. Its structure is constantly being reshaped, with new nerve cell connections forming according to our patterns of behaviour, emotion and thinking in the process that we call neuroplasticity.

While it is estimated that only 10 per cent of the activity of the brain is in conscious awareness, when we learn how to tune in with greater accuracy to our own emotions and the emotions of those around us, we are able to work much more directly with the activity of nerve cell circuitry and hormones that underpin our experience of life.

Whenever we are caught up in our heads, with our minds operating on autopilot, our brains work like a powerful simulator, replaying situations from the past and imagining experiences in the future which have not yet happened. When these simulations happen, the very same circuits of nerve cells and secretion patterns of hormones and neurotransmitters occur as if we were actually living the experience. A simple example of this is that if you were to think now of your favourite meal, what it looks like and how it smells, it is highly likely that saliva would start to flow and your stomach might start to rumble as it anticipates the process of digestion.

Let's see if we can use the power of our imagination to get a feel for how the emotions of others affect us. What we are going to do is imagine an interaction with a stranger and then with someone you know. It can be helpful for this exercise to set aside a few minutes when you won't be interrupted.

First, read through the script that follows and, if possible, remember the broad outline of the story and the steps involved in the reflection after each of the three scenarios. Sitting or lying down, with your eyes closed if it's comfortable, try to imagine yourself in the following story.

Experimenting with emotion

Imagine you are in a large department store. You are speaking with a shop assistant about returning a piece of clothing that you found didn't fit well when you brought it home. The shop assistant seems not the least bit interested in your situation and, looking at you with a scowl on her face, she says in a rather dismissive way, 'We don't exchange or return. Read the sales docket more carefully next time.' Then she turns to serve the next customer.

Pause now for a moment, and shift your attention away from the images in your mind, and any thoughts you might have. Turn the focus of your attention to any sensations you notice in your body and the pattern of your breathing. Can you notice tightness in any muscles, perhaps around your shoulders, back or face? Is there any discomfort in your chest or abdomen? What about your breathing—is it slow and steady, or more shallow and irregular? Simply note what you find. If possible, can you put a name to any emotions you feel? Take a few slow and steady breaths and then move on to the next part of the exercise.

Now imagine that it's the end of that same day, and you are seated with your partner at the dinner table. You're still feeling a little unsettled by what happened earlier and you decide to talk it over with them. They seem preoccupied, and as you are part way through telling your story, their mobile phone sounds that a message has arrived. They pick it up as you continue talking and turn to read the message.

Now let go of these images and, as you did before, take 20 to 30 seconds to allow your awareness to move through any sensations in your body, and take note of the pattern of your breathing. Once again, are you aware of any emotions or feelings that you can put a name to? Now take a few more slow and steady breaths, and move to the final part of the exercise.

This time, imagine once again that you are seated with your partner over dinner. As you begin to tell your story, they seem to pick up that you appear upset. Their eyes meet yours and you feel that you have their complete attention. Their phone sounds, but this time they quickly apologise and say, 'Let me turn that off.' They listen patiently without interrupting. When you are finished, they look at you with a concerned expression and say kindly, 'What a dreadful day you've had! I can understand why you'd be rattled by that. Can I help in any way? Perhaps we could go back to the shop together on the weekend and speak to the manager?'

Again, let go of any images in your mind, connect with your body and breath. What do you notice?

Reflection

When you reached the part of this exercise where your partner began interacting with their phone instead of paying attention to what you were saying, can you recall an urge to do or say anything in response?

Our reactions to facial expression and tone of voice occur almost instantaneously and well beneath conscious awareness. This means that before we even know what is happening, it is likely that the content of our own thinking will be influenced by the emotions of the other person, picked up by the mirror neurones in our own nervous system. The more we pay attention in interactions to any information that might help us see more clearly the emotional experience of the other person, the less likely it will be that we get caught up in an automatic process of reactivity.

As you will come to understand when we explore this in later chapters, recognising and finding names for different emotions is now regarded as an important part of the process of building emotional connection (or attunement) in relationships. But this takes practice. It can be more difficult to label emotions than you might think, especially as there is often more than one emotion present at the same time.

One way of practising this skill is by putting a label on any emotion or feeling that you notice when you are interacting with another person. It can also be useful to make a mental note about why you are choosing that label—is it a facial expression that you have noticed, or a tone of voice, or something else—perhaps the way the interaction has made you feel? We can easily make assumptions about the emotions of others. In the first scenario described above, when you imagine speaking with a shop assistant, you might label her emotion as 'angry'. However, we are not really able to know what is actually going on for her. Perhaps she is a mother with a sick child, and she is worried and preoccupied with this, and frustrated with your question. Being curious about emotion can help broaden our understanding of all that might be contributing to a situation and our reaction to it. ■

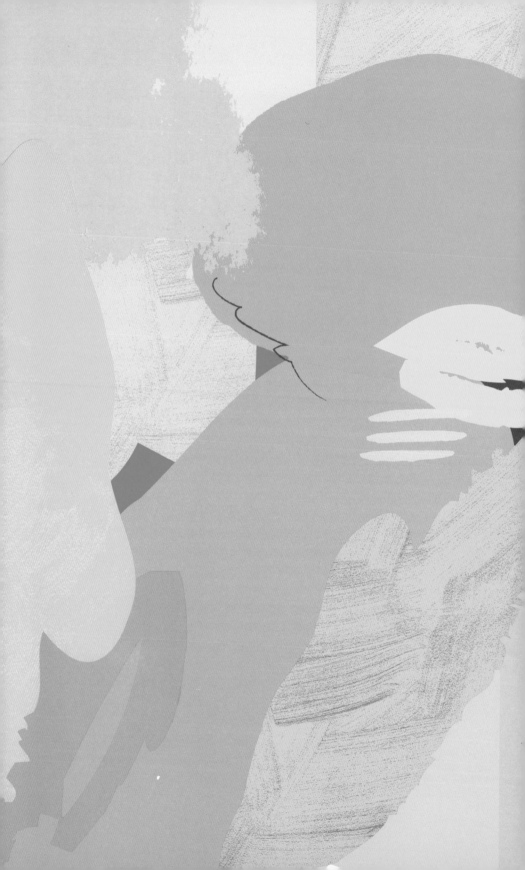

Stress, strive or connect — the three main circuits of emotion

E motions are at the very heart of what gives our life meaning, but, as we all know, they can wreak havoc, when without permission they sweep in and take over how we think and behave.

Sunila's story

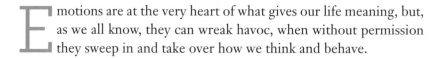

Sunila had just taken her daughter Gemma to her classroom and was about to take two-year-old Matthew to crèche. It was Gemma's first day of primary school and she had been anxious and reluctant to go. Matthew had sensed that his mother was distracted and in recent days he had wanted more of her attention too.

Having settled Gemma into the classroom, Sunila noticed as she turned to leave that Matthew had begun playing with toys in a corner. She was running late for work, so taking Matthew's hand, she tried to lead him out of the room to get to the car.

But Matthew was absorbed with what he was doing and had no intention of leaving. 'No, not going!' he cried as he lay down on the floor with one of the toys. Sunila felt embarrassed in front of the teacher and other parents. Kneeling down to his level she quietly but sternly said, 'NOW, Matthew; Mummy needs to go to work. Come right now!' But Matthew was determined, and as Sunila tried to gently pull on his hand, he started crying, kicking his legs and hitting out with his arms. This was now too much for Gemma, who had been trying hard to be brave, and she ran to her mother in tears.

Let's face it, it's not easy to prepare for the challenges parenting can bring! Ordinarily Sunila was a gentle, perceptive mother who was sensitive to the cues of her children, but when Matthew started screaming she felt as if all eyes in the classroom were on her. She was feeling embarrassed and exposed, assuming that the others were judging her as a mother. All she could think of was how she could get out of the situation as quickly as possible.

At another time, when she felt less uncomfortable, Sunila would probably have used an altogether different approach with Matthew when he began behaving in a way which, after all, was not at all unusual for a toddler. But on the first day of school, Sunila was keen to make a good impression with Gemma's teacher and with the other parents in the room. Powerful emotions like shame, anger and fear often take over when we are least prepared for them, robbing us of an opportunity to respond to what's happening in a calm and wise way.

Under the influence of the stress response and the rapid release of cortisol that comes with it, our brains respond as if a control switch has been flicked off and skills like insight and wisdom become unavailable to us as our frontal lobes go 'off-line'. The work of Professor Paul Gilbert, a research and clinical psychologist, has been particularly useful in helping us understand more clearly how emotions have evolved for specific purposes. They influence our behaviour in ways that have been crucial for our survival as a species, but unfortunately they can also cause us (and those around us) unnecessary pain.

Professor Gilbert's clinical work and research has helped clarify and distinguish the way that emotions can be broadly categorised into three main 'systems'—threat or stress, striving and pleasure, and finally the connecting and compassion system. When emotions get activated, specific nerve cell pathways light up, just like lights on a Christmas tree. With their cell bodies located in the brain, long connections run all the way down through the spinal cord connecting to our heart, lungs, gut and muscle tissue. As they become activated, specific hormones and a large number of different chemicals called neurotransmitters are secreted into the blood, around muscles, heart and gut and also into the cerebrospinal fluid surrounding the brain cells.

The threat or stress system is the most powerful. It is always running quietly in the background, never entirely switching off. It monitors our internal and external environments for anything negative or unwanted. From an evolutionary perspective, the purpose of this system was to protect us from danger. But for those of us who live in relatively safe environments, the triggering of this system happens most often in situations where we are reacting to an experience we would prefer to avoid, or, even more often, to difficult memories or worries about something which may or may not even happen.

When the threat system fires up, the level of the stress hormone cortisol increases instantaneously. When cortisol rises we feel stressed in our minds and our bodies. Our minds become highly active and our thoughts get hijacked by the issues that are causing us concern. Thoughts tend to race in a chaotic way, making it very difficult to think clearly. Interestingly, in humans the level of cortisol is at its highest around 4 a.m., which accounts for the fact that if we wake up in the early hours of the morning and something has been worrying us, it can be difficult to settle back into sleep.

Anxiety, irritability and anger are the most common stress-based emotions. In any given moment, the emotions we experience will influence the thoughts we have, how we feel about ourselves and how we behave. They can even affect what memories we have access to, which can be very problematic.

The second most powerful system of emotion, especially in Western society, is the striving and achieving system, and we can feel pretty good when this system gets activated. A chemical within the body called dopamine gets secreted and can lead to a 'high' much like people get when they use stimulants like cocaine or amphetamine. Like the threat system, the striving system has an important role to play, helping us get what we need to survive (and perhaps a little extra!), and achieve in important areas of our life. But these emotions which can start off giving us the enjoyable feelings of pleasure and success can end in a frantically driven state, where we are chasing goals, judging whether or not we are meeting our expectations, and in the meantime becoming more and more disconnected from the present moment.

The relative strength of various emotions depends on how often they are used. It's quite simple: the more often we 'practise' anger, striving, anxiety, irritability or worry, the stronger they become.

The most fragile and easily disrupted system of emotion is the safe, contented and connecting system. When this system is strong and healthy we feel safe, calm and settled, and we are able to see more clearly what is actually happening in the present moment, without the pressure of needing things to be different. Even in situations which are difficult, if we manage to activate the safe and connected system, we don't detach from the challenges we face; in fact, we see clearly what is happening. But we are able to respond from a more wise, balanced and caring position.

Like everything else in our nervous system, the relative strength of various emotions depends upon how often they are used. It's quite simple: the more often we 'practise' anger, striving, anxiety, irritability or worry, the stronger they become.

This bias in favour of threat- and achievement-based emotions over kindness, courage and wisdom is not our fault. We are built from the genes up in a way that has us exquisitely sensitive to threat (even if it's only our own worried thoughts) and searching for ways to acquire things that we think will make us happy—a new car, a glass of wine or, in Sunila's case, a well-behaved toddler!

Coming back to Gemma's first day at school, when Matthew decides to ignore his mother's request, we might imagine that anger and embarrassment would be the emotions that Sunila will feel. When her 'anger circuit' lights up, Sunila is more likely to remember all the times she has struggled with Matthew's behaviour, rather than the times when things have gone well. She might think, 'I'm sick of this naughty behaviour. He's always such a difficult child. Why can't he be more like his sister?' Matthew would see a completely different 'version' of his mother—the version that appears when he doesn't do what she asks. From the expression on her face to the tone of her voice and the way she behaves—all will feel different to him.

While it is not our fault that our brains are hardwired to be more sensitive to negativity, if we want to have warm, stable and healthy relationships then we need to learn how to address this bias.

Reflection

When you feel anxious, frightened or angry are there any typical ways in which you see yourself or how you are as a parent or partner? ◼

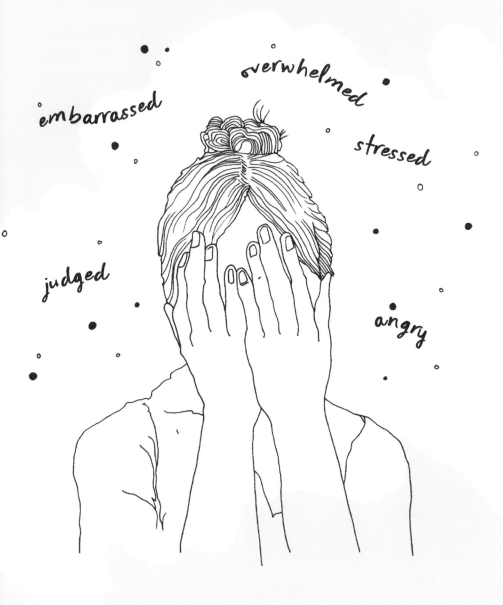

The tunnel vision of negative emotion

Connections
and disconnections
in families

Connections and disconnections, feeling heard and understood one moment and not the next. This is the dance which is constantly going on in our relationships. At times we hardly notice it's happening, but at other times we are painfully aware of it. In our important relationships these disconnections can get so big that they behave like blindspots—potholes of reactivity we fall into with concerning predictability.

A couple's story

As Nina sat before me I could sense her despair. She and her partner Ian had been on a long journey of IVF treatment for infertility, and the process had been exhausting and stressful. After two years there had been no pregnancy, and Nina was wondering whether it was time to give up on their dreams of having a child.

As hard as this was, what concerned Nina even more was the impact that the two years of treatment had had upon her relationship with Ian. 'We used to be so good together; I don't know what's happened. He's not interested in how hard this has been for me; he just says he's sick of how emotional I get. I really don't know if our relationship can survive this. Mostly I don't mention it anymore, but when I do try to talk to him about how I feel, he just shuts me down.'

It's very easy to take our relationships for granted, assuming that intimacy and connection should somehow happen without any special effort. But operating on autopilot in relationships is quite a risky business. If we are distracted and preoccupied, it is likely that our reactions will be influenced not only by expectations of what should be happening, but by invisible templates from the past.

Each time Nina and Ian ended up with a painful disconnection in their relationship, it felt more difficult to get out of. No doubt they were under a lot of pressure, but there is more going on here than meets the eye. Understanding this less visible dimension of reactivity that almost all of us have in relationships (our own personal blindspots) opens powerful opportunities to build strength and stability that had not previously seemed possible.

The clue to these underlying and often unhelpful patterns usually lies in experiences we had many years earlier, as children and adolescents—what is technically called our 'developmental history'. This forms a crucial part of every psychiatric assessment because it gives essential information about our underlying personality, our areas of relative strength and vulnerability. Much like finding missing pieces of a jigsaw puzzle, these insights can guide us to new understandings and fresh perspectives from which we can design constructive ways to move forward.

To understand this a little more clearly, let's take a look at what emerged in the developmental histories of Nina and Ian.

Nina grew up as the eldest of three children, in a close family that was loving and supportive. But Nina's mother was quite an anxious and timid lady. She worried a lot about the health of her children, and tended to race them off to the doctor at the first sign that they might not be well. Nina didn't doubt that her father loved her and her two sisters, but he was often loud and irritable and had no patience at all for his wife's worries. Nina grew up very accustomed to the loud arguments her parents had, and remembers many times when being at home felt like she was walking on eggshells.

Nina didn't know too much detail about Ian's childhood, except that both his parents had busy professional lives and had encouraged their son to be independent and study hard, which was exactly what he did. What Nina had noticed was that despite the journey she and Ian had experienced with IVF, her parents-in-law never really asked how things were going. In fact, they seemed unaware of how stressed their son was, and Nina didn't feel at all comfortable speaking to them about the concerns she had.

When her threat system was activated, Nina had virtually no access to more sophisticated intellectual skills of clear thinking and creativity.

What I hoped for in taking this background history was to find a slightly different way of understanding this young couple's relationship difficulties, and this is the hypothesis I came up with.

Nina had grown up to be a young woman very focused upon her physical health; probably with a heightened awareness of body sensations. The IVF interventions often caused her to have pelvic discomfort and tiredness, so it was no surprise to me that from the beginning of the program, she was very preoccupied with trying to make sense of her various aches and pains. Compounding this, I suspected that Nina found it challenging to deal with conflict in her relationships. Despite their best intentions, Nina's parents had not equipped their daughter with skills enabling her to be calm and balanced when she was upset, and assertive when it was needed. Years later in her marriage, whenever Ian raised his voice or seemed at all dismissive of her concerns, Nina's experience was of being shut down.

Taking Ian's formative years into consideration, coming from a family which did not really communicate at all about their emotions, it was not hard to imagine that Ian may well have felt ill equipped to deal with his wife's emotional demands. What happened when Nina tried to communicate her distress to Ian was that both of their 'threat systems' lit up. As we have learned, with each emotion we have there tend to be specific thoughts and storylines that come with it, as they are hardwired together down in the limbic system. When Nina and Ian were enjoying time together watching a movie or chatting over a meal, Nina felt loved by her husband, and was able to think beyond their current difficulties. However, when she became distressed and worried about the unsuccessful and expensive fertility treatment, and it seemed that Ian was not interested, different circuitry determined how she felt about her relationship. At these times she became convinced that Ian really didn't care too much about her. She even thought that maybe it was not a bad thing that they hadn't managed to get pregnant—how on earth would they cope with being parents together? When her threat system was activated, Nina had virtually no access to more sophisticated intellectual skills of clear thinking and creativity, the very tools required to step out of the limited storyline that determined the way she responded. In fact, each time Nina and Ian found themselves in their respective 'black holes', neuroplasticity ensured that it was more likely they would find their way back there again.

Nina and I worked together over the next few months using techniques of mindfulness to help her learn how to react less strongly to difficult emotions—either her own or those of the people around her. With practice, Nina learned how to bring more curiosity and interest to the role that emotion was playing in how connected or disconnected she felt in the moment. From this more neutral position of observing, Nina was more able to think clearly and be skilful with what she said. Rather than upsetting him, when Nina learned how to express herself in a more composed and calm way, she found Ian much less defensive. In fact, it became clear just how much he wanted to get close to her but being overwhelmed by emotion himself, it had all been too hard.

Sometimes challenges like this can be like a blessing in disguise. For Nina and Ian, soon after they withdrew from the IVF treatment, Nina spontaneously fell pregnant. The hard work they had done on their relationship allowed them to manage the demands of pregnancy and parenting in a more collaborative way, with much more confidence and skill.

Reflection

When you look back on the experiences that you had as a child growing up in your family home, can you recognise any predictable patterns of how people dealt with strong negative emotion? Did anyone become angry and loud, and if so can you recall how that made you feel? Or perhaps in your home difficult emotions went underground, leaving everyone feeling as if they were walking on eggshells trying to avoid an explosion. If so, how did that make you feel?

Can you see any connection now between the models of communication you grew up with and how you manage strong emotion in your relationships as an adult? ■

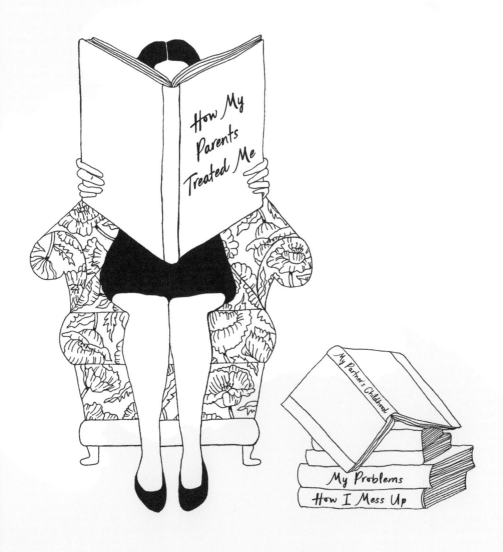

Our personalities are strongly influenced by our upbringing

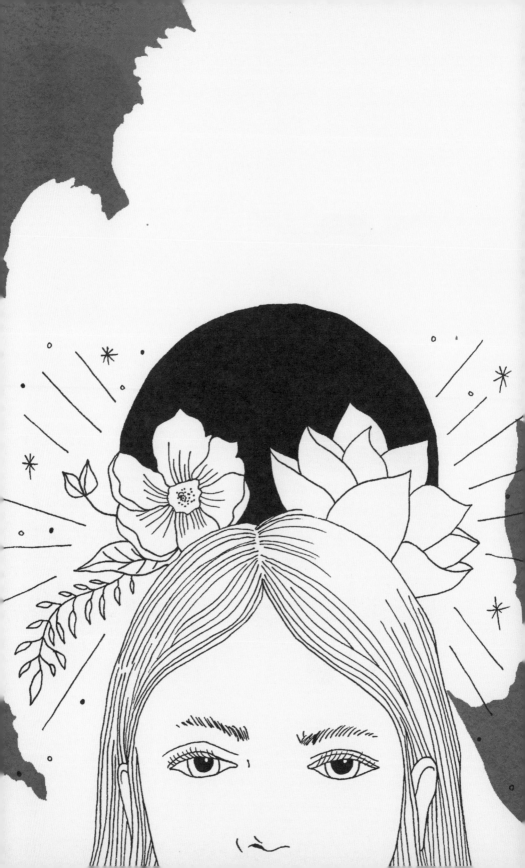

Part Two

PRACTICES AND TECHNIQUES TO TRY

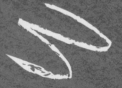

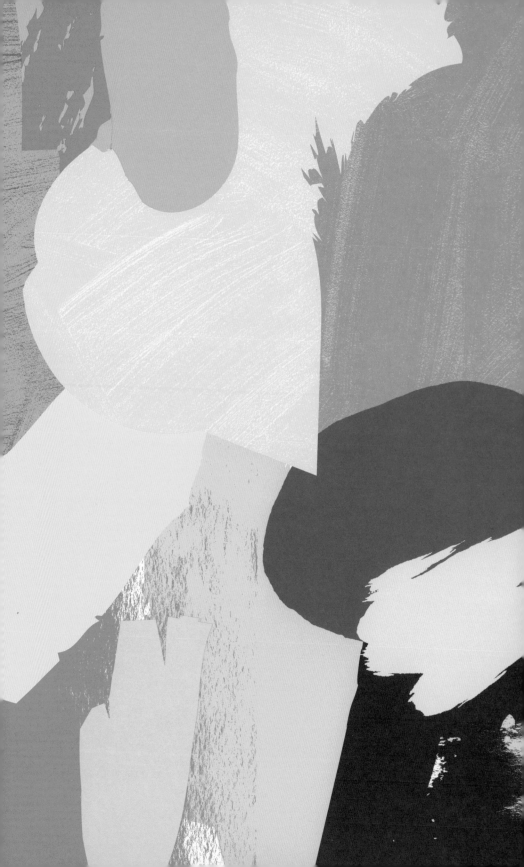

Lesson
6

Meditation — a personal practice

People decide to explore mindfulness for all sorts of reasons. For some it is the experience of anxiety or depression that awakens a desire to be more actively and directly engaged in the process of recovery. For others there is simply the dawning of a realisation that they no longer want to just exist in life, hoping that things will get better in the future. They want to get more out of life.

The concept of growing in strength and wisdom in the face of life's expected and unexpected challenges is what I observe over and over again when I watch young parents bringing techniques of mindfulness into their lives. A transformation takes place as they learn to not turn away from what causes confusion or pain. They come to embrace their difficulties with courage and stability, and by learning how to be fully present they often experience a shift in perspective, enabling them to respond with more creativity and skill.

Mindfulness is free, it doesn't require any special equipment and it can be practised anywhere. Whenever we remember, at any point in time, it's possible to step out of an automatic pilot way of experiencing life, to inhabit the present moment more deeply.

Mindfulness is simple, but not always easy; however, that's not because the techniques are complicated. There's a good reason why as humans we are so addicted to distraction and substances which promise short-term escape from the behaviour of our tricky minds. It can be relatively easy to be present and engaged in a moment when we are comfortable with what is happening—the laughter of a child, the tender smile of a friend, or simply the warmth of the sun on a cold winter day. But as we all know, to be fully present can also be hard—just imagining the cry of a baby, the tantrum of a toddler or the angry remark of a partner can be enough to send ripples of uncomfortable reactivity throughout our bodies and minds.

Mindfulness is free, it doesn't require any special equipment and it can be practised anywhere ... at any point in time, it's possible to step out of an automatic pilot way of experiencing life.

Mindfulness training in the form of meditation builds the nerve cell circuitry that provides the capacity for a steady and focused mind, the qualities that are essential if we want to bring a more creative and wise response to inevitable and unavoidable times of difficulty. Meditation has been used for centuries by people from all contemplative traditions, including Buddhism, Judaism and Christianity, as a means of stabilising the activity of the mind.

Mindfulness teachers often recommend preparing a place in the home for a concentrated meditation, where there's less likelihood of interruption. Some even find it helpful to drape a special shawl around their shoulders or light a candle as a reminder of the honourable tradition of using meditation as a way to meet what is difficult in life with fearlessness and an open heart.

Posture is important too. Lying down can be a good way to meditate at certain times, but might not be the best choice when you are feeling tired because it's easy to fall asleep. Mindfulness practice is very different from resting. While it is ideal to be able to relax into the practice, we are actually aiming for alert attention to whatever arises. Adopting an erect and dignified posture with the shoulders rolled back can also help by creating a spirit of openness and confidence, a sense of being ready to meet whatever arises.

In mindfulness training programs, participants are taught a range of practices, some as brief as three minutes. Practising any of them on a regular basis will be helpful. In general, the longer the practice the more likely it will be that challenging experiences will emerge— uncomfortable body sensations, difficult emotions and unwelcome thoughts, which is why the guidance of an experienced teacher, particularly early in the process of training, can make all the difference. But perhaps not surprisingly, the longer we practise, the more skilled we become at simply observing discomfort. Sooner or later as this capacity for observation grows, we come to experience a place of inner quietness, which many meditators come to regard as an inner place of refuge. A refuge that is not a place of escape, but rather a quiet and safe position from which a bigger picture or a more grounded understanding of what is happening becomes available.

As neuroplasticity embeds the process of mindfulness into the hardwiring of our nervous system we begin to notice that even when we are not meditating, there is a new default system. A greater awareness of the activity of the mind is available to us, and gradually we become less likely to act impulsively or to get hauled into loops of negative thinking. As this process becomes automatic we begin to feel as if finally we are in the driver's seat of our life.

In Lesson 1 we met Jonathan, who was experiencing low mood and anxiety after the birth of his second child (see page 19). When I first saw him, the extent of his irritability and the difficulty he was having with memory and concentration had me initially thinking that he might require a combination of antidepressant medication and mindfulness training. However, after spending time in our first session helping Jonathan understand the impact that sleep deprivation and stress was having upon the workings of his brain and how mindfulness training might help, he told me that he was keen to postpone the use of medication and see whether he might be able to bring about change himself by dedicating time to a daily meditation practice.

Each week I set homework for Jonathan. I asked him to make space for twenty minutes each day for a formal meditation practice. When he returned to his appointment in the following weeks we discussed any difficulties he had encountered and what he might have observed.

While it's not clear from the research to date just how much time is needed in a formal practice of mindfulness to achieve a benefit, in my experience the significance of Jonathan's symptoms suggested that if he did not dedicate enough time each day for the exercises, he would be unlikely to experience benefit.

In the following two chapters you will find descriptions of a few of the foundation meditation practices commonly used in mindfulness training programs. When first learning how to meditate, it can be helpful to be supported by listening to a recorded meditation, and in the Resources section at the end of this book you will find a list of websites where you can freely access recorded meditations.

Reflection

Perhaps you are considering developing a mindfulness practice for yourself. Are you clear about what your motivation is? What might be different in your life if you could bring greater focus, insight and even courage to what is happening?

In previous chapters we have been exploring how tricky minds are, and how easy it is to turn, as Jonathan did, to distraction or keeping busy in an attempt to deal with the busy mind. Have you tried to bring a practice of mindfulness into your life before and found it frustrating or difficult? What sense do you make of that? ■

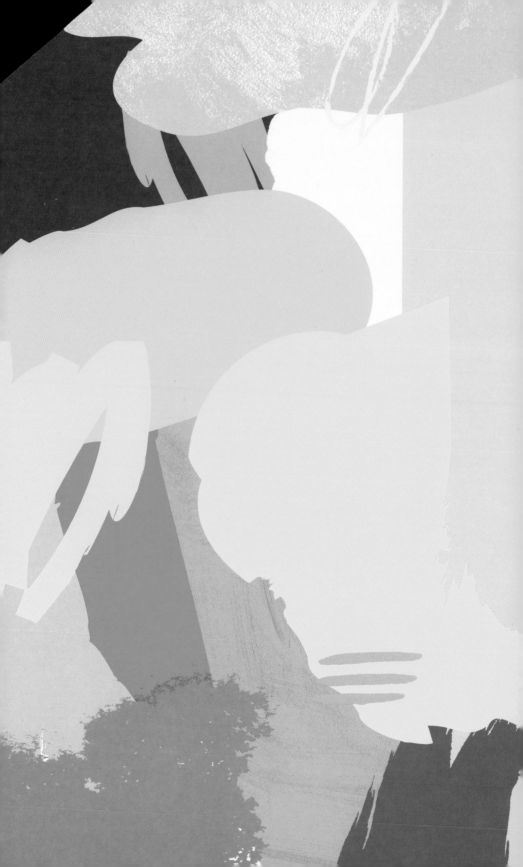

Lesson 7

Meditation — body-based practices

The purpose of meditation is not about trying to change anything. We simply learn how to direct the focus of our attention in specific ways. The focus of attention is the muscle we aim to strengthen. We expect that thoughts will arise, sometimes there will only be a few, but more often there will be many and at times they are likely to feel strong and compelling. The heart of the meditation practice is noticing thoughts as they arise, and patiently and gently returning the focus of attention to the task.

When you listen to recorded meditation practices you may notice that the words 'gently' or 'kindly' tend to be repeated on a regular basis. The intention of this is to remind ourselves again and again to let go of judging what we're doing, or of driving ourselves to achieve a particular goal. As Jonathan had observed, there was already plenty of that going on in his inner world, and far from being helpful, he found that it simply served to disconnect him from the present moment and drive him more strongly into further thinking and planning.

Body scan meditation

Make yourself comfortable, either lying on the floor or on your bed, or sitting on a chair if that's what you prefer. Remind yourself that the intention of this practice is to bring careful attention to whatever is happening; not to try to make things different from how they are, nor strive to feel more relaxed or calm.

Allow your attention to rest for a few moments with any feelings you can notice in your body, perhaps the sensations of where your body meets the floor or the chair.

Now bring the focus of your attention to the area of the lower abdomen, becoming aware of any sense of movement associated with the breath flowing in and out of the body.

Imagine that this focus of attention can be like a spotlight which you can direct. Allow the focus of your attention to move all the way down your left leg to the left foot. As best you can, pay attention to any sensations that are present in the toes; perhaps there might be a tingling, or warmth or moisture. Or there may be no sensations, and that too is completely normal.

Keep in mind that it is in the nature of the mind to think—so it is bound to happen a lot and is not a sign that you are doing anything wrong.

Now see if you can imagine the breath entering through your nose or mouth, passing through the chest and abdomen down into the left leg, the left foot and then out to the toes of the left foot. On the following out-breath, imagine letting go of the sensations in your toes as the breath moves all the way up through the left leg, the abdomen and chest to leave the body through the mouth or nose. As the next breath enters your body, see if it's possible this time to bring awareness to the sensations in your left foot, simply being curious about whatever you feel. Once again, as the breath leaves your body, let go of the sensations in your left foot.

Following the movement of the next in-breath in a similar way, allow the focus of awareness to pass through your body, this time all the way down into the lower part of your left leg. Notice any tendency to 'think about' this part of your body, and as best you can try to simply tune in to any physical sensations that are present. On the following out-breath, allow the focus of your awareness to leave that part of the left leg.

In this way, on each successive in-breath, allow the focus of your awareness to move systematically through the body, gradually working your way through the left leg, then moving to the right leg, the pelvic area, the back, the chest, then both arms, neck, head and face. Simply allow each in-breath to guide you into the neighbouring area of your body in a gentle exploration of physical sensations.

Once you have finished scanning the entire body in this way, allow yourself to be aware of any sensations which come to your attention, and perhaps imagine that the breath can flow freely in and out, bathing the whole of the body with a calm and nourishing energy.

As with any meditation, there is no right or wrong way to do a body scan. Each time you manage to notice that you have been distracted, perhaps by thoughts or sounds, congratulate yourself. This capacity to notice and work skilfully with distraction gets to the very heart of a mindfulness practice.

After his first week of practice at home, Jonathan reported noticing what most people struggle with when they are first learning to meditate. 'I just couldn't stop my mind. I kept thinking I can't be doing this right; isn't this supposed to be making me feel more relaxed?'

A look of surprise came across Jonathan's face when I congratulated him. It was clear to me that he was doing the work I had asked of him, and it didn't surprise me at all that he was feeling confused. Remember, 90 per cent of the brain's activity is going on beneath conscious awareness. It's just not possible to turn thinking off, and in the early days of learning mindfulness it's important to be reassured that the point of the practice is actually to notice the activity of the mind and to redirect the focus of attention. We become so used to being totally caught up in the activity of our minds or trying to distract ourselves that we are often unaware of how challenging it can actually be to anchor our attention in what is actually happening in the present moment.

In Jonathan's second week of practice I suggested that he alternate his daily body scan with some mindful stretching.

Mindful stretching

Stand in bare feet or socks with your feet a hip width apart, and your feet more or less parallel to each other.

On an in-breath, slowly raise your arms out to the sides, parallel to the floor, and then after breathing out, on the next in-breath slowly raise your arms until the hands reach high above your head. As your arms move, see if you can be fully alive to the sensations in your muscles as they work to lift the arms and then maintain them in the stretch.

Allowing your breath to move in and out at its own pace, continue to stretch upward, with your fingertips gently pushing towards the sky, your feet firmly grounded on the floor. Once again take time to feel the sensations of the stretch in the muscles and joints of your body.

When you are ready, on the next out-breath, slowly lower your arms until they rest beside your body. Feel the changing sensations as they move, noticing perhaps the feeling of your clothes as they move on the surface of your skin.

With the next in-breath stretch each arm and hand up in turn as if you were picking fruit from a tree that's just out of reach. Notice the breath as you look up beyond the fingers. Allow the opposite heel to the outstretched arm to come off the floor as you stretch, feeling the sensations through your body, from the fingers of one hand to the toes of the opposite foot.

As you return your arms to your side, tune in to how it feels to let go of the effort that is required to lift the weight of each arm.

And finally now, play with rolling your shoulders while letting your arms rest by your side. Begin by raising your shoulders upwards towards the ears as far as they will go, then roll them backwards, as if you are attempting to draw the shoulder blades together, then allow them to lower completely. Now squeeze your shoulders together in front of the body as far as they will go, as if you were trying to touch them together.

Allow your breath to determine the speed of rotation. Continue rolling through these various positions as smoothly and mindfully as you can, first in one direction then in the opposite direction.

Whenever you find yourself carried away by the intensity of physical sensations, or by thoughts, feelings or daydreams, gently reconnect with the here and now by refocusing your attention on the movements of the breath or on a sense of your body as a whole.

Connecting to body movement and sensations is an important part of mindfulness training. The importance of body-based practices has been known for centuries in many cultures and in traditions such as yoga, tai chi and aikido, which have been regarded as powerful means of restoring emotional balance and an inner sense of calm.

As modern neuroscience has begun to investigate the connection between body sensations and emotion it has become very clear that our bodies quite literally hold emotion. Whether it's the uncomfortable sensation of not being able to get enough breath when we feel anxious, or the tightness in the muscles around our face when we're worried, body-based practices are now understood to increase the strength of hardwired nerve cell connections to the central nervous system or brain.

With practice we become more sensitively attuned to sensations in our body, which in turn gives us direct information about our emotions. Over the weeks that followed the beginning of his training, as Jonathan got more experience with body scanning and gentle stretching, he started noticing that he was more aware of physical sensations, even when he wasn't meditating. 'One day it just seemed obvious to me as I walked through the front door that I had a frown on my face. Nothing too extraordinary about that, I suppose, but it made me stop and take notice. It occurred to me—what must it feel like for Katie and Thomas when the first thing they see when I arrive home is me looking worried or not happy.'

Jonathan was beginning to tune in to his emotions. This was giving him a precious opportunity to observe what was going on within and get a better understanding of what could be contributing to his experience of irritability at home. In that session, as we explored in more detail what it might mean to be able to notice the tension he was carrying, Jonathan began to talk about an evening a few days previously when, within ten minutes of walking through the front door, he found himself getting angry with Thomas. 'When I get home I feel like all I really need is some peace and quiet, and it's so hard when Katie just hands me Lyla and at the same time the TV is blaring away and Thomas is racing around the house making a loud racket. I feel so bad about it now, but when Thomas didn't listen when I asked him to quieten down I just yelled at him and told him to go to his room.'

In our work together we were beginning to get access to the difficult experience most parents feel at one time or another, when exhaustion leads to a reaction which only serves to further escalate tension and unhappiness. 'I remember the night so well, and it's not easy for me to talk about it. I felt frustrated with Katie that she didn't understand that I too had had a hard day, and I suppose I was feeling angry. But then when I yelled at Thomas it was as if it was just too much for me and I couldn't seem to get back to a more calm state. I knew that what I was doing wasn't helpful but I just couldn't think clearly.

'I can see now, Thomas was just wanting my attention. I really want to do better as a dad.'

Reflection

How aware are you of sensations in your body? How do you know when you feel tired, stressed, angry or happy? When we use these labels, it is the physical sensations that we are actually referring to. Next time you become aware that you are putting a label upon how you feel, see if it's possible to quickly scan through your body and describe more clearly what physical sensations are present. ■

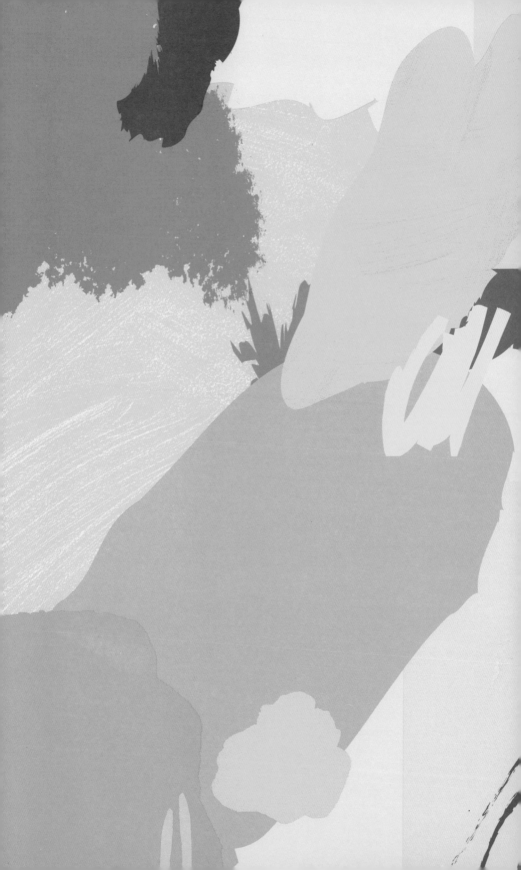

Meditation— breath practices

W hen scientists began exploring the traditional technique of breath meditation, it was never anticipated that they would find it to be a powerful practice impacting directly and immediately upon the function of both our bodies and minds.

Research conducted by Professor Richard Davidson has demonstrated how practising yoga breathing for half an hour a day for just two weeks changes the structure of the brain, and similar breath practices successfully treated young war veterans who suffered from previously treatment-resistant post-traumatic stress disorder.

Research from the University of Quebec revealed that there is a unique pattern of breathing for each different emotion we experience. These scientists also showed how we can generate any emotion including fear, anger, joy and happiness by adopting the breathing pattern which is hardwired to that emotion. The extent to which the autonomic nervous system is balanced in a healthy way can be reliably measured by calculating whether the heart rate varies between the in-breath and the out-breath. This measure is called 'heart rate variability' (HRV). Low HRV is associated with impaired immune function, increased incidence of heart disease, and stress-related illness such as anxiety and depression. HRV can be measured quite easily with the use of mobile phone apps that utilise the phone's inbuilt camera.

As we have been learning, whether something is happening in the present moment which upsets or frustrates us, or whether we are simply caught up in a pattern of worried thinking, the stress response kicks in automatically, beneath conscious awareness. The stress response instantaneously recruits activity in a system of nerve cells which runs throughout the body and brain. Called the 'autonomic nervous system', there are two main parts to this network of nerve cells connecting our brain to our heart, blood vessels, muscles, skin, gut and lungs.

One component of the autonomic nervous system is the 'sympathetic nervous system', which is responsible for the stress response. When it gets activated the level of the stress hormone cortisol rises and the network of nerve cells distributed throughout the body prepares us for a fight, flight or feint response. Although we may not usually give it a name, if we are paying attention we can feel in our body when the sympathetic nervous system gets activated. Our muscles tense, our heart beats faster and it can be hard to think clearly.

The 'parasympathetic nervous system' is the other 'arm' to this nerve cell network, and it is responsible for the body's inbuilt relaxation response. It lowers the heart rate and blood pressure and allows for more nourishing blood to get to the frontal lobes of our brain, which in turn gives us access to the more sophisticated processing functions of creativity, lateral thinking and abstract reasoning.

In Lesson 4 we looked at the three main systems of emotion, and the consequences of the fact that as humans the threat and striving systems tend to be much stronger than the nerve cell networks that allow us to feel safe and connected. Anxiety, anger and irritability are the most common emotions associated with the threat and striving systems, and the research into neuroplasticity tells us that the more we practise emotions, the more strongly they get embedded within our nervous system. For Jonathan this meant that the more practice he got with irritability and anger, the more likely it was that those emotions would show up again.

Over the next few weeks Jonathan began alternating each day with a mindfulness of the breath practice and a body-based practice.

Mindfulness of the breath meditation

Come to a comfortable position sitting on a chair with your feet flat on the floor, and gently close your eyes. Allow yourself to tune in to any sensations you can notice in your body, remembering that there is no need to change anything, or create a particular type of experience with your mindfulness practice.

Direct the focus of your awareness to any sensations you might notice deep in the abdomen. Is it possible to pay attention in such a way that you can notice the gentle flow of the movement of the breath as it enters the body through the nose or mouth and passes down into the body?

If you notice that your mind is particularly busy, it can be helpful to place one hand flat on your abdominal wall and pay attention to any movement you can feel when you draw attention in this way to the changing pattern of sensations.

Once the focus of your attention has steadied and you are able to notice the movement of the breath, you can remove your hand and focus more closely on sensations of the breath in the abdomen.

As with any meditation, you may be distracted by noises or thoughts. This is perfectly normal and is bound to happen a lot, so it can be very helpful to practise congratulating yourself for being so aware of what's going on.

As best you can, imagine that it might be possible to simply allow these distractions to be there, without needing to change anything, while you patiently return the focus of your awareness to the movement of your breath.

Continue this way for ten minutes, or more as time permits, gently reinforcing an intention to quietly observe the steady movement of the flow of breath in your body.

There is a brief adaptation of the breath meditation, called the breathing space practice, or the STOP practice (see the exercise that follows). It was designed specifically to be portable, and to help bring mindfulness into the experience of day-to-day life. In fact many people who participate in the eight-week training programs come to find this to be one of the most important things they learn. To get a feel for how this practice can be helpful it is usually suggested that you schedule a three-minute breathing space practice on a regular basis, two or three times throughout the day.

For Jonathan this worked best when he was about to take a break from his work at morning and afternoon tea time and before lunch. Working in an open-plan office, Jonathan found that by continuing to appear as if he was working at his computer, it was possible for him to move through the three steps of this brief practice without anybody around him being aware of what he was actually doing.

Breathing space or STOP practice

The three steps of this brief practice have been likened to the image of an hourglass, with the focus of attention being broad in the first and last minute of practice, narrowing to follow the movement of the breath in the second of the three minutes.

Step 1: Awareness

Coming to an upright and dignified posture, bring your awareness to all that you can notice in your inner world. Note the presence of thoughts and, as best you can, try simply regarding them as temporary experiences that come and go. Next, see if it's possible to identify any feelings or emotions, and if you can, put a brief name to them like worry, happy or sad. Finally, briefly scan your body for any physical sensations, making a note of any tightness or discomfort.

Step 2: Gathering attention

In this step we gather up the focus of our attention in such a way that it can rest more directly on the sensations of the movement of the breath in and out of the body, wherever it is most easy for you to feel. This might be where the air enters through the nose or mouth, or through movement you notice in the chest or the abdomen. When possible, allow a full minute to patiently redirect the focus of your attention away from any distracting thoughts to the sensations of the movement of the breath.

Step 3: Expanding awareness

Allow the field of your awareness to expand now to take in all the sensations that are present in your body as a whole, including the sense of your body's posture and your facial expression. If you become aware of any experience of discomfort, see if it's possible to imagine that the breath could move in and out of this area allowing a softening and relaxing around the sensation. Again, allow a full minute to develop this feeling of expanded awareness.

You might find it helpful to use the term 'STOP' practice for this exercise. The letters of this word describe another way in which the brief practice can be used:

S—Stop what you are doing.
T—Take a few deep breaths.
O—Observe your experience: thoughts, body sensations
    and emotions.
P—Proceed, taking with you a memory of what it really feels
    like to slow down and observe what is happening.

This breathing space practice can be one of the most effective ways of stepping out of automatic pilot mode, or of lessening the grip of difficult emotions.

Jonathan found that in his third week of using this brief practice, there were unscheduled occasions when it occurred to him that it might be helpful to use the technique. Even when he didn't have the full three minutes available, he found that going through the individual steps, however briefly, seemed to really improve his capacity to recognise what was going on for him, and in doing this he seemed better able to reconnect with the present moment in a less distracted way.

By now you may have come to understand why building insight is considered to be one of the most significant benefits of a mindfulness practice. For Jonathan, as his practice of mindfulness consolidated, insight came in the form of how he was experiencing the most basic of day-to-day occurrences:

'Before I learned how to use mindfulness I thought I would never be able to get used to how tired I always felt, and how resentful I could get when one of the children disturbed my sleep. Now it's as if I am still very aware of the sensations of feeling exhausted, but I choose not to buy into them in the same way, and I especially watch out for those really unhelpful thoughts about why I'm not getting enough sleep, and the tendency to blame someone, which only causes me to be more unhappy than I need to be.

Building capacity to be really present to what is happening in the moment, without allowing the activity of the mind to be hijacked by unnecessary thinking, can lead to significant improvement in mood and quality of life.

'I've also noticed that I feel so much better since I put limits around getting on my phone or answering emails when I'm at home. It's been really helpful to just put my phone and laptop in the study whenever I'm at home. Depending on what issues are happening at work, I usually allow myself half an hour max in the evenings to go in and check whether there have been any important messages or emails that I need to respond to. The rest of the time actually feels calmer to me. It's easier for me to see now how carrying my phone around when I'm at home made me feel as if work was right beside me all the time. If my boss SMS'ed me—well, I may as well have been back at work. For at least a few minutes my head would be totally disconnected from being present with Katie and the kids.'

Jonathan's experience with mindfulness is a good example of how building capacity to be really present to what is happening in the moment, without allowing the activity of the mind to be hijacked by unnecessary thinking, can lead to a significant improvement in mood and quality of life. When Jonathan originally came to see me and expressed his desire to try to manage his symptoms of depression with mindfulness alone, I was happy for him to give it a go, but his irritability was so prominent that I thought it might be too hard for him without the initial assistance of antidepressant medication. He proved me wrong and I really admired his self-discipline and the patience he found for his practice.

What might also have been helpful was a discussion that we had in our first session about ways in which he could more directly experiment with shifting emotional states. As Jonathan was already very aware of the impact that his irritability was having at home, I suggested that as often as he remembered, he practise talking more slowly and quietly than he ordinarily would as a way of bringing attention to his style of interacting. I also suggested that Jonathan experiment with imagery as a way of counteracting the negative thoughts he was having about his relationship with Thomas. I thought it might be helpful for him to specifically recall a memory of a good time he had had with his son, then bring an image of this experience to life in his mind on a regular basis and as vividly as he could.

After some practice with this, Jonathan found that paying attention to an image of Thomas that he created in his mind could help him get in touch with warm feelings for his son. He found that if any self-critical thoughts arose he simply noted them and returned the focus of his attention for a few more moments back to the image.

Within the first month or two, Jonathan's dedication to the process of learning mindfulness had paid off, and a significant improvement in his mood occurred. One of the early and most striking changes that he noticed was his ability to let go of irritability. Then, without any specific direction from me, Jonathan came to discover for himself how he could use time with Katie or either of the children as an informal way to practise. Jonathan's strong motivation to connect more warmly with his family allowed him to see that by paying careful attention to what was actually happening in the moment, simply being with Katie or either of his children could be an opportunity to practise letting go of thoughts and connecting more directly with his family.

Reflection

Perhaps Jonathan's story has made you wonder about how the informal practice of mindfulness might provide you with an opportunity to work more skilfully with experiences that might otherwise contribute to stress.

Reflecting upon the routine of your day-to-day life, can you think of any situations that tend to predictably contribute to tension, which you could target with informal mindfulness, and perhaps use a three-minute breathing space practice in the way that Jonathan did? ■

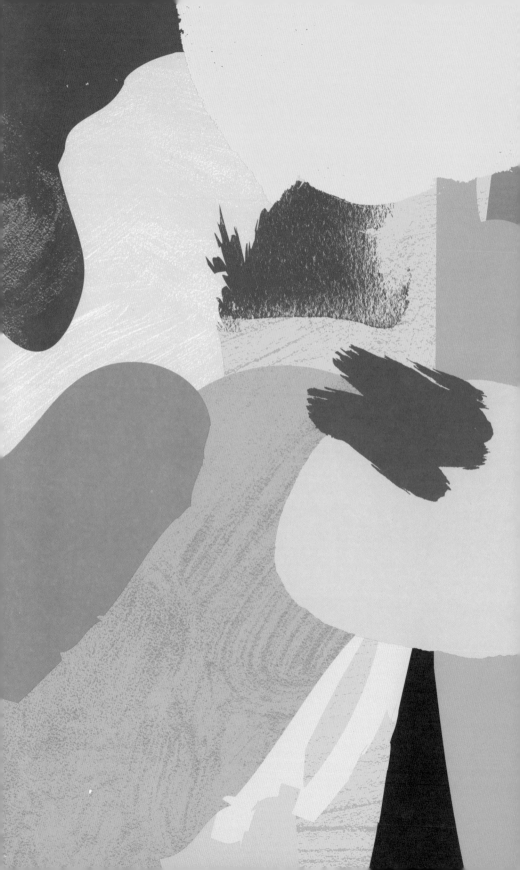

Lesson 9

Formal and informal practices

Mindfulness teacher and psychologist Jack Kornfield,
referencing American author Anne Lamott

When we are disconnected from what is going on around us, and caught up in a pleasant daydream, mind wandering can feel quite enjoyable; like a welcome distraction, especially when the reality of the present moment feels uninspiring or worth avoiding.

Yet in an instant this pleasant little reverie, fuelled by the pressured momentum of our own thoughts, can without our permission haul us in to a less reassuring inner dialogue. Disconnected from the present moment we become vulnerable to the influence of feelings such as worry, fear, irritability or anger. These emotions impact upon how we see ourselves and our life, but they also affect what we bring to parenting and to other important relationships.

Sarah's story

Sarah had been diligently practising mindfulness for two years and came to see me because she was disappointed with her progress. She was clearly very motivated to take care of herself physically and emotionally. She went to a yoga class three days a week and the other days made time to sit quietly on her own and follow recorded meditations on an app on her mobile phone.

'I'm not sure how mindfulness is supposed to work,' Sarah said. 'I like doing the meditations, and for a little while I feel more relaxed, but the rest of the time, I'm just as irritable and cranky as ever. The effects just don't last.'

Sarah explained that she had a high-pressure job and the culture at work was not particularly healthy. Over the years she had been with the organisation, morale had steadily fallen. There had been ongoing funding cuts and management had been ruthless in letting go of staff.

When she was at work, Sarah was usually distracted by worry about whether her job was secure, and what she would do if she was asked to leave. When she was at home she remained irritable and preoccupied, and her two adolescent daughters seemed to be picking this up and had become tense and unsettled too.

Sarah's experience with mindfulness is not at all unusual. Research reliably shows that when well understood and practised regularly, significant changes in brain structure and function are measured in only eight weeks. Keeping this in mind, it therefore seemed likely that there were critical aspects to the use of mindfulness which Sarah did not understand.

Meditation is really only a means to an end. While it can be a very helpful way to build mindfulness skills, many people don't understand how to integrate what they learn into daily life. Despite her yoga and meditation, Sarah had little understanding of how her mind was reacting to the issues which caused her stress. The way that Sarah had been using an app to assist her meditate was at best probably only building concentration and focus. At worst, it might have been functioning as an escape—a quiet time away from life's demands, with the words of the guided practice acting as a distraction.

The Buddhist teachings upon which mindfulness programs are based have as a core intention the development of insight and wisdom. There is no attempt to suppress thoughts; in fact, it is in the very noticing of the activity of the mind that we come to build insight into why we might be struggling in certain aspects of life.

With training we can build strength in areas of the brain which are habitually underutilised. You might decide to learn how to play a musical instrument, and by practising regularly specific areas of the brain which have little to do with thinking would become larger and stronger. In much the same way, if you were interested in building deeper and more emotionally connected relationships, it would help to take mindfulness skills into your interactions with others. You would then be building strength in the circuitry of the brain involved in communication. With practice you might more sensitively 'tune in' to what is happening in your interactions and be less likely to respond in ways that are not well thought through.

... it is in the very noticing of the activity of the mind that we come to build insight

So how does mindfulness practice work? Right now your brain is processing millions (quite literally) of pieces of information simultaneously—from your five senses, from sensations deep within the body and muscle tissue, and also the flow of thoughts as they emerge. Obviously it's not possible to be aware of all this information at the same time, so deep within the brain there is a strong filtering process going on.

Stress occurs when the negativity bias of the powerful threat system impacts upon the filtering of information in such a way that thinking and ruminating reduce our ability to be aware of most of what is actually going on in the present moment.

The eight-week formal mindfulness courses are carefully constructed. For example, the meditation on body sensations (called the body scan) helps anchor attention far away from thinking, and as we tune in more accurately to body sensations, we become more aware of changes in our emotions. As we shall see in Lesson 10, breath meditation is a portable and powerful practice which gives us the capacity to directly feel and work with the body's stress response. These are examples of formal mindfulness practices.

Informal practice is when we bring focused attention to other activities. Let's see how Sarah did this.

Sarah's progress

In her new formal practice, Sarah completed a twenty-minute body scan on alternate days. After listening to the recorded instructions a few times, she practised on her own.

While this was initially quite challenging, Sarah could tell that it was a much more effective way to learn. Without the distraction of the audio guide, Sarah was left alone with the activity of her mind, and she had to take responsibility for noticing when her mind wandered, and return her attention again and again to the body scan.

In her regular yoga class Sarah also paid more attention to what her mind was doing, and where in her body she noticed stiffness and tension. In between classes she made an effort to 'drop into' how her body was feeling—stretching or adjusting her posture when needed.

As an informal way of extending her practice, Sarah began paying particular attention to what was going on in her mind when she was at work and with her family. She monitored more closely the activity of her mind, and whenever she noticed that she was distracted she brought the focus of her attention back to the task at hand.

Sarah particularly wanted to change how stress was affecting her home life, so as she travelled home by train each day, instead of distracting herself by reading or checking emails, she chose to sit quietly, simply watching all that went on around her. While doing this she softened into any muscle tension and gently encouraged her breathing to be a little slower and deeper. Each time thoughts about work came into her mind, she redirected the focus of her attention back to the present moment.

Just as every moment in our life is different from the last, each experience of mindfulness will also be different from any other. Sarah had found a way to strengthen her practice and adapt it in such a way that it was of practical use to her outside times of formal meditation.

Reflection

Have you ever noticed how an experience of feeling stressed can affect your interpretation of what is happening in the present moment? For Sarah, her busy, distracted mind affected many ways in which she experienced life at work and at home, and it is no surprise that she found great benefit in bringing techniques of informal mindfulness to her interactions at home with her children and at work with her colleagues.

Have you noticed any predictable ways in which stress impacts unhelpfully upon important aspects of your life? Can you think of ways in which you might be able to use informal mindfulness to help? ◼

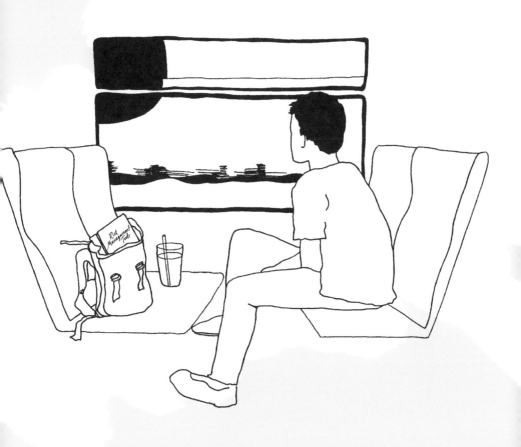

Focus attention on enjoying the present moment without distraction

Lesson
10

Just this breath

Breath practice is the perfect way to take the power of mindfulness with us into every part of the day. It is beautifully portable and as we discovered in Lesson 8, it is especially useful as the breath is intimately linked to the very foundation of the stress response.

Professor Paul Gilbert has coined the term 'soothing rhythm breathing' for the style of slow, steady breathing which extends deep into the abdomen, shifting the autonomic nervous system into a relaxation response.

As with any mindfulness practice, our aim is to patiently return the focus of our attention again and again to the anchor we have chosen. Noticing when our attention has wandered is the first essential step in building the muscle of mindfulness. But trying to concentrate on the movement of the breath can be harder to begin with than you might think.

Soothing rhythm breathing practice

For this exercise it can be helpful to be in a quiet place, away from distraction. If it's comfortable, sit or stand with your eyes gently closed.

As best you can, pay attention to the natural rhythm of your breath as it moves in and out of the body. You might notice a sense of coolness as the air passes into your nostrils and warmth on the exhalation. Or perhaps it's down at the abdomen, where you can feel a slight up-and-down motion as the breath enters and then leaves the body.

See if it's possible to comfortably slow down the pace of breathing so that on each in-breath and out-breath you can count silently to five. If this presents any difficulty then don't persist; perhaps simply reconnect with a sense of the breath movement at its own pace while also paying attention to the feeling of being grounded with your feet firmly on the floor.

Allow this soothing rhythm pattern of breathing to continue for another couple of minutes, then widen the focus of your awareness to take in sensations in your body, and then an awareness of your physical surroundings. Gently open your eyes.

Leah started seeing me twenty weeks into her third pregnancy. She had a history of depression which had started in adolescence, and had used antidepressant medication for most of her adult life. It had been her hope to stop the medication before she fell pregnant, but whenever her dose was reduced she became irritable and her sleep deteriorated.

So with the intention of trying to take a more active role in her emotional wellbeing, Leah had begun doing some excellent work with a psychologist, and she had also started attending a local meditation group. When she first came to see me, Leah was confused by the difficulty she was encountering with the mindfulness practices, which she had expected would help her relax.

Leah's story

'Whenever I try and focus on my breath, it's as if my mind goes wild. I feel even more anxious and I think I'm never going to beat this, and if I can't manage this, how on earth will I cope with a baby.'

As Leah was discovering, when we try to turn the focus of our attention in a direction of our choosing, what we inevitably encounter is not just the busyness and chaos of a multi-tasking mind, but often also a negative commentary running away in the background. When she tried to focus on her breath, Leah was getting a very close look at how the circuitry of irritability and self-criticism worked within her.

This is why it's essential to pay attention to the spirit or emotional tone we bring to the practice. The more we can be playful and gentle rather than trying to force things to be different, the more effectively we will be able to bring about positive change in the complex fabric of our mind and body's stress response.

As I worked with Leah we found ways to begin to weave in more gentle and supportive self-talk and feelings. As it turned out, Leah often tried to practise when she felt she needed it most, when she felt at her most stressed, so it didn't surprise me that she was having difficulty.

I asked Leah to spend a few moments before she started her breath meditation, connecting to her body with some gentle stretching. I also suggested that rather than sitting to do her breath meditation, she might try standing, and adjusting her posture so that her shoulders were rolled back, her spine was erect and she was able to get a good feel for the movement of her breath from the tip of her nose, through her chest and deep down into her abdomen.

I asked her to soften the muscles around her face and shoulders, and bring a slight smile to her face as if she was welcoming her life-giving and nourishing breath.

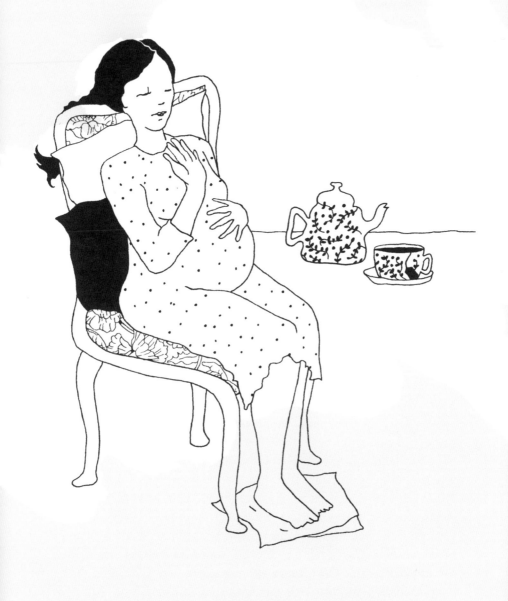

Breath meditation is a powerfully effective and portable practice

I then asked Leah to practise guiding herself quietly with some simple words spoken in a warm and supportive tone. On the in-breath she would say, 'Just slowing my breath', on the out-breath 'Slowing my mind'. Each in-breath and out-breath would be slow and steady, lasting for about five seconds each.

Leah began each day with fifteen minutes of this breath practice, and later when she was sitting on the train on her way to and from work, she found she could allow her gaze to rest on a book on her lap, and again connect to slow, steady breathing, supported by the words she had practised, this time spoken quietly in her mind.

This practice Leah took with her throughout the day. As with any mindfulness practice, our goal must be to integrate the skills into everyday life. When Leah first came to see me, it was at work that she most noticed stress taking a toll on her emotions. Despite her long history of depression, Leah's symptoms had been well managed with the use of antidepressant medication; she had coped well after the birth of her first two children and subsequently with the demands of work and family life. But it seemed that from the beginning of this third pregnancy, feelings of frustration and irritability had been difficult to manage. Leah worked in a busy department store as a sales assistant, a job she had really enjoyed up until the last year, when staff shortages meant that customers often had a long wait to be served and understandably became frustrated or angry.

As Leah became more confident in her mindfulness of breath practice, we focused on helping her connect to an awareness of her breath to help slow down her mind and settle her emotions when she was caught up in stressful situations at work. As we have been learning, mindfulness give us a capacity to *be aware of* and *observe* what is happening in the moment. As confidence in her skills improved, I suggested that Leah actively look for situations when her customers seemed unhappy or dissatisfied. Using her heightened ability to observe her breath, she noticed that at those times she was often barely breathing! Her body was tense and the little air that came and went from her body moved only into the upper part of her chest. Although it was initially challenging, Leah came to see that it was possible to soften the tension she felt in the muscles of her shoulders and face, and, at the same time, to deepen and slow down the pace of her breathing. With practice she found that she could do all of this while remaining closely connected to the interaction she was having with her customer. In time she found that the greater sense of inner calm that she experienced seemed to silently soften the experience for those around her.

Paying attention to her emotional tone, as she was learning to do, she began to find that she could drop into a completely different emotional space wherever she found herself. Whether she was at work or doing household chores, Leah found a much greater awareness of the pattern of her breathing, which she eventually used in the labour ward to provide a stable anchor when she was giving birth to her daughter.

Reflection

Tuning in to our pattern of breathing can be a powerful way of finding out more about our emotions. Try seeing if it's possible to identify different rhythms of breathing that seem connected to your own emotions—pleasant and unpleasant. With which emotions do you notice your rate of breathing is more rapid or shallow? ■

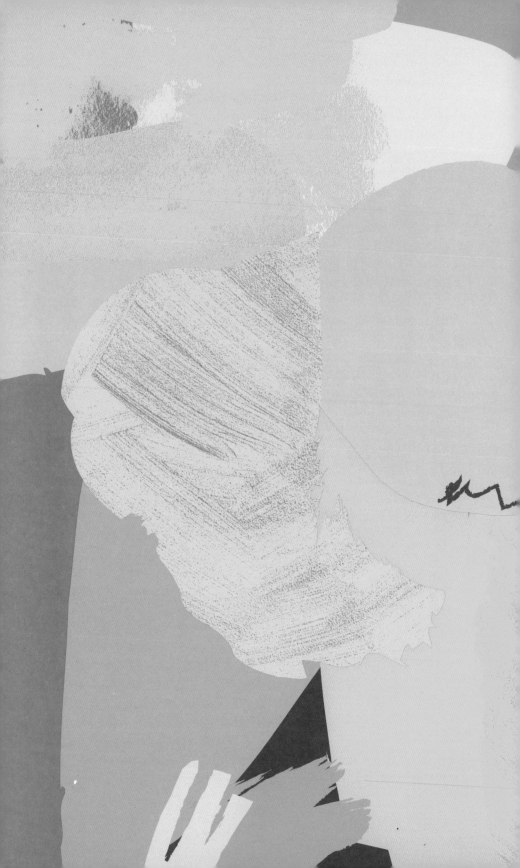

Inhabiting the body

E motions are quite simply sensations in the body which become hardwired to particular patterns of thinking and behaving. In fact, research has revealed that just as each emotion is linked to a unique pattern of breathing, so too are different emotions associated with particular body sensations and postures.

The body scan and walking meditations are foundation practices in mindfulness training for a number of reasons. From a practical perspective, turning the focus of attention towards body sensations is a straightforward way of disconnecting from the flow of mental activity. But in addition to this, research shows that regularly tuning in to body sensations creates greater nerve cell connections between the body and the brain, which in turn leads to the hardwiring of emotional resilience. The technical term for recognising the physical sensations connected to emotion is 'interoception'. Generally when strong negative emotion arises it takes a while before we recognise what is happening because we get lost in the storyline.

Before we know it we can be caught up in a powerful flow of negative thoughts, and potentially react in unskilful ways. Bringing the focus of attention to body sensations (as we do in a body scan) increases the number of nerve cell connections from the body and muscles to the area of the brain which registers sensation.

Susan's story

Life for Susan was frantic and rushed. Worries about work and money were on her mind most of the time. She and Jim had two young children and she said that she'd never anticipated how difficult it would be to juggle all the demands of family life. She felt disconnected from her two daughters, and she said that her two-year-old's behaviour was becoming hard to manage.

'I'm so irritable. In the evening I can't wait to get the children in bed so I can unwind in front of the TV, but then I feel guilty. It's not the sort of mother I want to be. My husband reacts to my snappiness by just going quiet, and takes off into his study.'

Within a few minutes of beginning her first session with me, as she began to tell her story, I observed a total transformation in the way Susan presented. When she initially entered the room she seemed quite bright and confident. Dressed in smart business clothing she presented as articulate and composed, and for a few minutes I felt puzzled about what the purpose of her visit might be.

But as she began to tell her story, there was a dramatic change. Susan's posture slumped in the chair, she lost eye contact with me, and her voice faltered as tears fell. I took advantage of the sudden shift in emotion to introduce a brief mindful exploration.

'Susan, I wonder if we could just slow this down for a moment. It's taken a lot of courage to be as open and honest as you've been, and we can learn a lot from what is happening here in the room. I'd like to see if it's possible for you to connect with any sensations you have in your body. Is there anything you notice, any muscle tension, or physical discomfort?'

'I feel a heaviness in my chest; it's hard to get my breath and there's a tightness across the back of my shoulders.'

I led Susan through a brief mindfulness practice, helping her direct the focus of her attention away from the storyline which was impacting so strongly on her emotions.

A brief mindfulness practice

If it feels comfortable, gently close your eyes. Sitting comfortably in your chair but with an erect posture, allow yourself to connect with the sensations you might be able to feel in your body.

Note any thoughts and as best you can try to simply let them go. Allow the focus of your attention to now go to the sensation of the movement of your breath as it enters and leaves the body at the nostrils.

I'd like you, for a few moments, to bring the focus of your awareness to a very small area around your nostrils. Noises might still intrude, or thoughts might seem strong, but your practice is to see if it's possible to simply accept this and firmly redirect the focus of your attention again and again to the sensation of your breath as it enters and leaves the nostrils.

When you are ready, with your eyes still gently closed, see if it's possible to broaden the focus of your attention to take in any physical sensations in your body, and then expand to an awareness of the room around you.

Gently open your eyes. See if it's possible to take with you into the remainder of the day a greater awareness of the movement of your breath.

This was Susan's first experience of disengaging from the flow of her thoughts, and connecting more directly with the experience of emotion in her body.

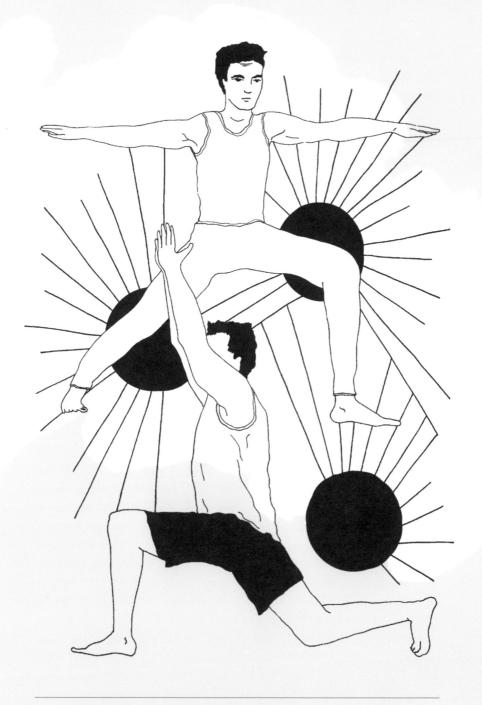

Exercise has a proven benefit to mood as well as to physical health

When we returned to the process of taking a history and exploring how life was for her, Susan was noticeably calmer and seemed more able to reflect upon all the things which might have contributed to the difficulties she faced.

Aerobic fitness and careful attention to our physical bodies has a lot more to offer than the widely accepted impact on our physical health. Regular aerobic exercise has been shown to release specific hormones and chemicals (endorphins and dopamine) that lift mood. In fact, in many cases regular physical exercise can be an effective alternative to medication in the treatment of anxiety, depression and other emotional disorders.

Over the next six months, Susan saw me on a regular basis. We explored the ways in which her habit of pushing herself hard and judging whether or not she was living up to the expectations she had of herself (and others) had contributed to her current symptoms of depression. As Susan built insight into the way her mind worked and how the pattern of her thinking could lower her mood and contribute to irritability and tension in her relationships, we began to tailor a mindfulness practice which would help her build emotional resilience.

Until she had her children, physical exercise was an activity that Susan had enjoyed. She used to swim and play tennis regularly, but since becoming a mother her exercise routine was, at most, a 30-minute jog a couple of times a week. For Susan, exercise had become a chore, another item on the to-do list. When she did go for a run, she put on headphones and tried to escape from her thoughts by listening to music.

Going for a jog was potentially a great way for Susan to improve her fitness and her mood, but we needed to find a way to enrich the experience for her, and I wanted to see if we could build it into a formal practice of mindfulness. We had already learned that Susan tended to hold a lot of tension in her body, and that she was quite unaware of the effect this was having upon her mood and thoughts. So to begin with, I suggested to Susan that it would be helpful if she could find five to ten minutes each day to practice mindfulness of the breath. This helped her learn how to observe what was going on in her mind, and enabled her to tolerate this awareness, and then to disconnect from the flow of her thoughts.

With the support of her husband, who minded the children, Susan set her morning alarm a half an hour earlier than usual on alternate days. This allowed time for a twenty-minute jog in the adjacent park before she got ready for work. Instead of her usual habit of listening to music while she ran, I suggested that Susan use the experience to practice noticing thoughts and reconnecting with a greater awareness of what was going on around her.

'I feel like I come to life when I run,' Susan said when she next saw me, a couple of weeks after beginning the new exercise routine. 'When I begin, my mind is usually noisy, and initially I really missed not being able to escape into the music I was used to listening to. But it didn't take long for me to see how paying attention to the sounds I could hear—the birds, the cars, the sounds of my feet as they hit the ground, can actually be quite relaxing. Then I began to notice that it could be a little while before I became aware that a train of thoughts or worry had pulled me in again. When I paid more careful attention to what was going on, it felt like I had tunnel vision—I was barely aware of what was going on around me. My shoulders were tense and my jaw was clenched. Initially this annoyed me, but now I find I can simply let go of the tension and reconnect to the world outside.'

Reflection

When we are disconnected from the sensations of emotion in our body, we are less likely to recognise how these feelings might be influencing our thoughts and behaviour. As Susan found when irritability was taking a toll on the relationships she had with her children, we may be more likely to behave in ways that are not wise as a consequence of this lack of awareness.

Become familiar with the 'signature' sensations of emotion in your body. Pay attention when you notice anxiety, irritability or anger—can you recognise patterns of sensations? Connecting to body sensations when emotions are challenging can also be an effective way of grounding the attention, allowing any strong emotion to pass before acting. ■

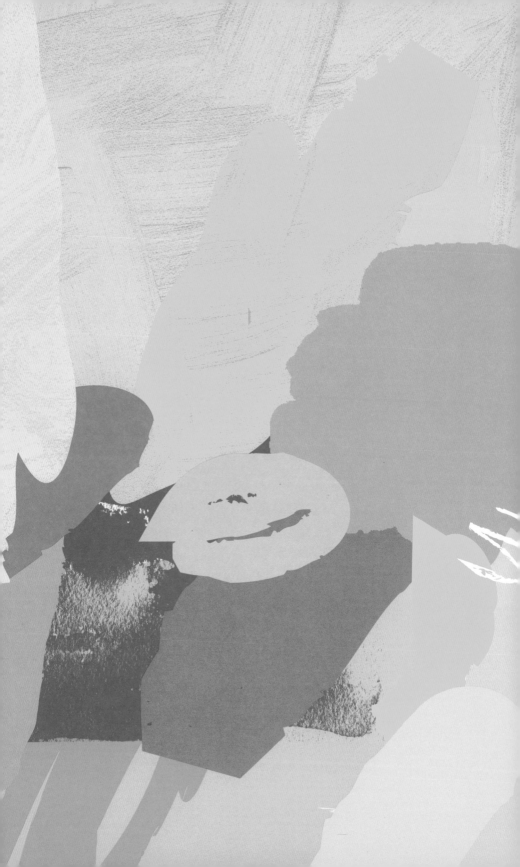

Lesson
12

Riding
the waves
of emotion

Emotions like fear, anger or irritability have a habit of erupting into our lives at the worst possible time, leaving a trail of chaos behind them.

No matter how much wisdom we might have after the event, when we are unprepared, a wave of strong emotion can haul us into a reaction that develops its own destructive momentum. Before we know it we may unleash an angry tirade of words that we later regret, or behave in a way that only serves to create greater disconnection in our relationships.

We can use mindfulness skills quite strategically, as a means of focused resilience training, specifically targeting the aspects of our life where we have developed strong and unhelpful patterns of reactivity. Mindfulness then becomes a way of riding these waves of reactivity, grounding us in the present moment and providing a space of awareness from which we are able to observe what is happening with more clarity and greater balance.

Edward's story

Edward initially came to see me concerned about how stress and irritability were creating significant problems for him at work. He explained that he and his wife Tamara had had Millie, their first child, eight months earlier. Ed said that it had been a challenging few months as Millie was not a great sleeper and was often unsettled during the day and the night.

Ed said that his stress had been getting a lot worse since he had begun getting up to the baby through the night so his wife could catch up on sleep. He had noticed that after his sleep was disturbed, his mind was usually very active, and it was difficult for him to get back to sleep. As Ed had become more tired, his capacity to focus and pay attention at work had deteriorated and his boss had begun documenting complaints about the quality of his work.

Ed was able to see that as he became more stressed he was finding it difficult to remain composed in conversations. Both at home and at work his irritability was taking a toll. Whenever his boss tried to give him feedback, Ed tended to react defensively and the conversations rarely went well. His local doctor had referred Ed to see me when his boss had delivered an ultimatum—to lift his performance and change his attitude or his position in the company would be reviewed.

One of the important ways in which mindfulness differs from other forms of therapy is that it teaches us how to disengage from the underlying storyline. Under the influence of stress, the processing of information in our minds becomes rigid rather than flexible, and we usually hold onto only one limited perspective of what is happening.

In our first session together, Ed's storyline was indeed quite fixed. He felt that it was very unfair that his boss didn't seem to take into account the fact that Ed's life was temporarily affected by the changes that had happened after the birth of Millie. Ed thought that all his years of loyal service to the company seemed now to be of no importance to his boss. In his home environment, Ed's tiredness and irritability resulted in him being preoccupied and distracted. While Ed had described Tamara as distant and low in her mood, it seemed likely to me that she might in part be responding to a difficulty in getting close to her husband.

As the first session drew to a close, I reassured Ed that what he was experiencing was incredibly common following the arrival of a baby. The huge transition to parenting and the tiredness that comes with it invariably makes it difficult to approach challenges constructively and creatively.

Our work together started with getting Ed back into an exercise routine. Regular aerobic exercise can be a powerful way of reducing stress. In addition to this we worked on helping him build a daily mindfulness practice. I taught Ed how to begin with a few body stretches then move to a ten-minute breath practice. When he was focusing on the breath, I suggested that whenever he noticed any distraction he simply label it, in whatever way felt useful, then patiently but firmly return the focus of his attention to his breath. Noticing the distractions was as important as being attentive to the rhythm of his breathing.

The huge transition to parenting and the tiredness that comes with it invariably makes it difficult to approach challenges constructively and creatively.

Over the next couple of sessions we addressed how Ed might look at what he found challenging in a more neutral way, much like he was learning in meditation, by simply noting any process of 'reactivity'. We started by making up a list of all the things he did on an average day which contributed to frustration or irritability. For homework, Ed was to take the list with him and pay particular attention to what was going on in his thoughts and body sensations when he noticed feelings of worry or irritability. I wanted to help Ed see more clearly what reactivity looked and felt like, before he became caught up in a story about it.

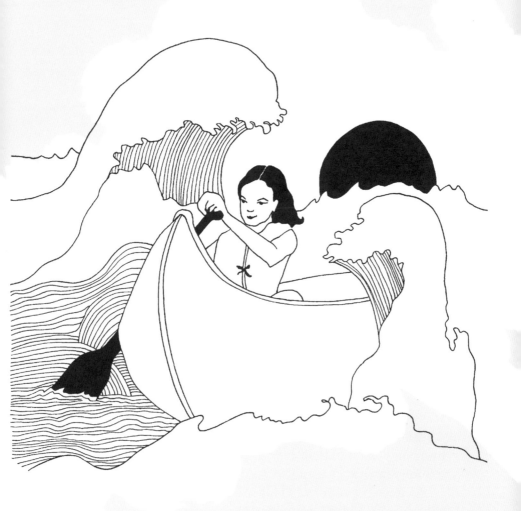

Mindfulness teaches us skills to ride the waves of reactivity

Edward's list of reactivity

What's happening	Reactivity
Washing the dishes at night	Frustrated and bored. Slight headache, sore shoulders
Standing in crowded tram	Annoyed with other passengers. Tension in shoulders and face
Hearing Millie cry at 2 a.m.	Sinking feeling in chest, weary, low mood
Noticing boss observing work	Hands clenched, feeling really annoyed, tempted to get angry with boss

In the next stage of his mindfulness training, I asked Ed to practise responding to reactivity by seeing if it was possible to simply reconnect to his breath. As best he could, Ed was to allow his breathing to become slower, deeper and more regular, extending right down into his abdomen.

The intention was for Ed to use an active process of mindfulness to disconnect from thoughts and reduce the chances of being hauled into an old pattern of reactivity. Slowing and deepening his breath was also a way of intervening directly in the physiological stress response in his body. Slow and steady breathing helps activate the body's natural relaxation response.

When we begin to use mindfulness to ride the waves of negative reactivity, it can feel as if we are just chipping away at layer upon layer of reactivity. Paying attention to reactivity when it showed up in his daily tram commute may not have initially seemed to Ed as related to handling a conversation with his boss, but it was actually an important opportunity for practice.

The stress response begins well below conscious awareness, deep in the limbic system, which means that all of the experiences of reactivity that Ed listed actually start in the same way, by triggering an initial response in the amygdala. This in turn leads to increased levels of stress hormone. As we have already learned, when cortisol rises, Ed's capacity to connect to frontal lobe skills was reduced, and he was no longer able to think clearly or be creative in how he responded.

Despite how it might feel in the heat of the moment, the natural life of any emotion is to simply rise up and then fall away within seconds. Research shows that even the strong and uncomfortable emotions like anger and fear only escalate within us when they manage to hook us into a reaction. That reaction may be a process of thinking or a way we behave.

When we begin to use mindfulness to ride the waves of negative reactivity, it can feel as if we are just chipping away at layer upon layer of reactivity.

Remember that emotions operate like electric circuits—when a circuit of sadness lights up, memories, images and stories that are linked to that feeling are automatically triggered. When we get angry in an interaction with someone, our reaction is going to be automatically complicated by memories of past occasions when we have felt that way. Sometimes we are aware of those memories, often we are not, which is why at times our reaction can seem out of proportion to what is actually going on in the present moment.

Reflection

Try using mindfulness as a way of noticing how negative reactivity impacts upon your life. As a way of prompting more flexibility, see if you can identify the storyline that comes with it. Remember that whatever your story might be in that moment, it can only ever be a small part of a bigger picture. Perhaps ask yourself, is this story helpful or not? Is there any other way I could look at this situation? ■

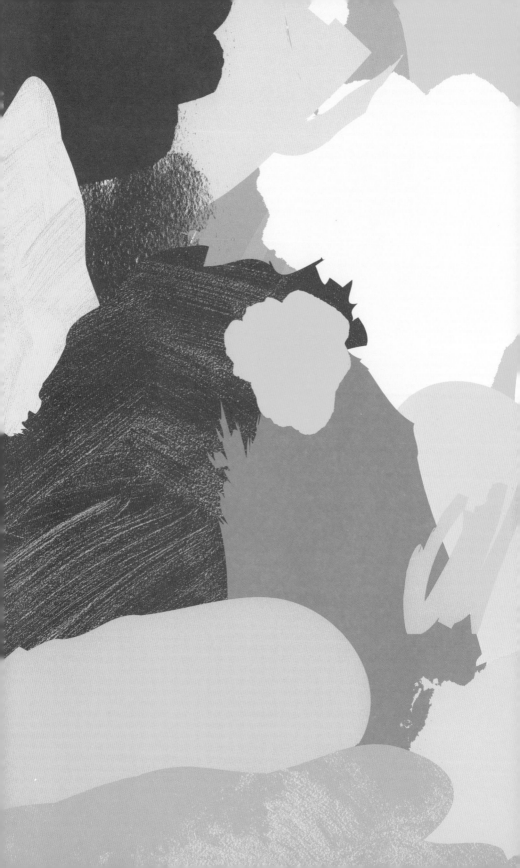

Lesson
13

A mountain of courage within

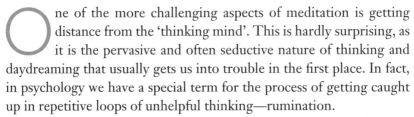

One of the more challenging aspects of meditation is getting distance from the 'thinking mind'. This is hardly surprising, as it is the pervasive and often seductive nature of thinking and daydreaming that usually gets us into trouble in the first place. In fact, in psychology we have a special term for the process of getting caught up in repetitive loops of unhelpful thinking—rumination.

In Lesson 1 we looked at the way in which the human brain is actually hardwired for negativity, with 90 per cent of the mind's activity being generated beneath conscious awareness. The consequence of this is that when we engage in a process of arguing with our thoughts it is very likely that the consequence will be to hardwire the process of rumination around that particular topic. The next time a similar thought emerges it will be more likely to reactivate the same unhelpful and repetitive inner dialogue.

In practising mindfulness we are not trying to create a refuge to hide away from the negative thinking, but we can still use the concept of a refuge to help us imagine developing an inner space of awareness which feels more neutral and welcoming. From this position of relative quietness, disconnected from the flow of thinking, we simply observe the activity of our mind.

Imagery can be a wonderful way of extricating ourselves from rumination and troubling emotional states like worry, boredom, fear and irritability, and the stories that accompany them.

Despite the ready availability of courses and teachers, many people struggle with mindfulness because what they encounter in the activity of the thinking mind can feel negative, fragmented and unruly. Professor Paul Gilbert suggests we experiment with antidotes to these challenges by doing what we can to bring a kind, playful and relaxed mind to our mindfulness practice.

We can be creative with a mindfulness practice, and imagery can be a wonderful way of extricating ourselves from rumination and troubling emotional states like worry, boredom, fear and irritability, and the stories that accompany them.

A traditional practice in mindfulness is the mountain meditation. Aligning ourselves with the qualities of majestic natural environments like the sea, the sky or a towering mountain can be a unique way to bring to life an awareness of the strength we can all find within.

You might like to read this script of the mountain meditation through once or twice, then find yourself a quiet place to allow the focus of your awareness to turn within. Set aside however much time you can allow or feel comfortable with. (You can find a recording of a mountain meditation on iampresent.com.au)

The mountain meditation

Find a comfortable position, preferably upright, but you could also do this meditation lying down. To this position bring a sense of dignity and commitment to be fully present and alert.

Allow your attention to rest with the sensations of where your body meets the floor or chair, and connect also with the feeling of your breath as it enters and leaves your body.

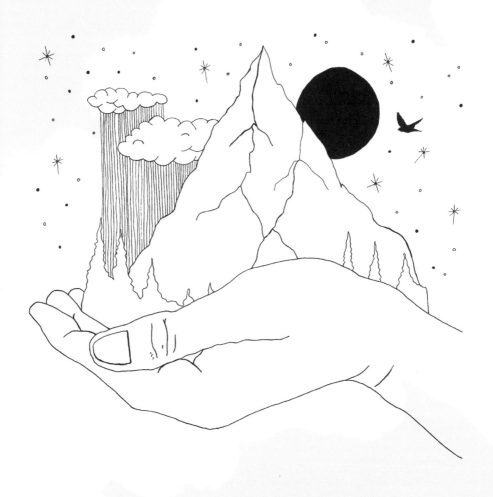

Mountain meditation

Let go of any motivation to create any particular change, just notice how your mind is at this moment, and perhaps find a word that describes it such as busy, calm, agitated or quiet.

Now bring to mind an image of a mountain, perhaps one you have visited, or seen in a picture, or simply one created in your mind. Allow this image to become clear, notice its size and shape as it stretches up high, all the way from the earth to the sky.

Bring awareness to its beauty and dignity.

Is your mountain topped with snow, or is it covered with trees?

However it appears, just allow it to be there, as you notice your breath moving steadily in and out of your body.

Allow yourself to become this mountain, strong and unwavering with its stillness, strength and beauty.

Birds might fly around it, clouds and storms will pass over it and seasons will come and go. Still the mountain remains just as it is, patient and wise.

Just like the mountain, we can endure periods of darkness and light, moments of sadness and moments of joy.

All experiences are to be encountered, allowed to be present, then to pass.

Mountains can teach us this wisdom and stability, and much more; we just have to listen.

Charlotte's story

Charlotte worked very long hours as a senior accountant in a large organisation. Her partner Pippa was four months pregnant with their second child. When she first came to see me two years after completing a Mindfulness Based Stress Reduction course, it became clear that her commitment to a daily body scan practice had improved her capacity to concentrate, as well as her quality of sleep, and her tendency to be anxious. Previous life experiences, however, had shaped Charlotte's personality in such a way that she was quite goal oriented and solution focused, which was not always helpful as a partner and parent at home where emotions often ran high.

Charlotte grew up as the eldest of three children, but her mother died when Charlotte was only ten years old. Her father was a tough man with a fiery temper who worked hard to meet the practical needs of his children, but it was left to Charlotte to become a surrogate parent to her younger siblings. She learned the hard way that to be strong was more comfortable than to be 'weak', and to push on and demand a lot of herself and her younger sisters was the most effective way of coping.

Her relationship with Pippa was a strong one. Together they had navigated the stressful path of conceiving two pregnancies with donor sperm and managing the reactions of extended family and friends. Mostly, Charlotte handled the tasks of parenting with skill and dedication, but that changed as Pippa's pregnancy advanced and she became overwhelmed with tiredness and prolonged morning sickness. It was Pippa who was generally more intuitively in step with the emotional needs of their son Ben, and Charlotte came to see how much she also relied upon Pippa's capacity for patience and kindness. As their family situation changed and Charlotte needed to step up in her ability to emotionally support both Pippa and Ben, it became clear that the mindfulness practice that Charlotte had initially found helpful had become another source of frustration.

'It's not working anymore,' was Charlotte's terse comment about her daily body scan. 'I can't even stand doing it anymore; it's easier to unwind by watching the TV.' Initially Charlotte seemed quite disconnected from her emotion. As she told me in our session about how life was going at home, she reeled off the various ways in which she had adapted her daily routine in order to meet the increased demands placed upon her by Pippa's tiredness. It occurred to me that something was missing in the story. I gently probed a little deeper. 'Charlotte, I wonder if perhaps there is something else about Pippa's tiredness and withdrawal that is worrying you?'

My question met with silence. For at least a couple of minutes I could see Charlotte fighting to remain in control of the situation. Then suddenly it was as if she collapsed from within. Her body bent over, she held her head in her hands and wept. 'I don't want her to die.'

My suspicion had been that Charlotte had never really had an opportunity to make sense of the premature death of her mother. Concealing her emotional vulnerability had not been a conscious decision, but a way in which her nervous system had learned how to reign in a very deep-seated loneliness and yearning for her mother.

It was time to build upon Charlotte's understanding and practice of mindfulness so that it might better address her own need to feel safe and capable of riding the strong waves of difficult emotion which needed to be processed. Charlotte came to find the mountain meditation immensely valuable. As she aligned herself with an image of a mountain and the feelings of having a strong and stable foundation, she allowed herself to feel that the challenging changes in the weather—the rain and hail and strong wind—were the sadness, fear and anger that emerged as she dared to acknowledge her emotions and memories.

Reflection

See if you can keep this image alive within you, as a way of connecting to this inner sense of refuge through day-to-day life. You might find it helpful to carry with you a small but special stone, which can be held whenever you want and act as a reminder of how the qualities of the natural environment can inspire and comfort.

The present moment can always be more than our thoughts and feelings. ■

The stories our emotions tell

Just like a fish caught on a baited hook, our minds get hauled into waves of reacting to emotion. Believe it or not, we can practise emotions! I wonder what might happen if you woke up one day and decided to devote the whole day to practising being angry. How do you think that day would work out?

That may sound a little ridiculous, but it's only because we become so used to being caught up in 'reactive' emotions that it is often not until long after a situation has passed that we are able to consider other ways of responding. At the time, the storyline that comes with the emotion is so familiar that we don't pause to consider an alternative interpretation.

A broken promise

Let's imagine that you wake up on a Saturday morning, looking forward to a morning walk and the warmth of spring. You had headed off to bed earlier last night to try to beat the first signs of a sore throat you had been nursing for a couple of days, leaving your partner in the company of a few friends who had come over for the evening. On waking you notice how quiet the house is. Your children and partner are still asleep.

'Time for me at last,' you think to yourself. You're looking forward to a brisk walk and think you might stop off for a coffee on your way home.

Walking through the lounge room, you notice glasses, an empty bottle of wine and plates with remnants of food on them; evidence of the evening before. Feeling frustrated and annoyed you head out towards the back door, thinking you'll get out for your walk and deal with the problem later. But as you walk through the kitchen more mayhem greets you. A carton of milk is on the kitchen bench, plates and pots and pans from last night's dinner remain untouched in the sink.

Now you feel angry. Your partner had sent you off to bed last night, aware that you'd had a big week and were not well. They reminded you that their friends were coming around but reassured you that they would keep the noise down and clean up all the mess.

'I am so sick of this,' you think to yourself. 'I can't rely on them to do anything they say they will. So much for a morning to myself!' Assuming that there is no way now that you'll be able to enjoy your walk, feeling resentful and angry, you set about tidying and cleaning up the mess in the kitchen.

As anger surges through you, memories from the past come tumbling into your mind, of other occasions when you have felt let down by your partner. Thinking of them still lying peacefully in bed, you might plan what you will say, how you will give them a piece of your mind.

How do you think the next conversation with your partner might go? We need to recognise these negative emotions when they arise, otherwise from deep within the brain in the part of the limbic system that files away memories and the emotions that go with them, a cascade of mental events gets triggered. Stories based upon experiences from the past merge with the current wave of reactivity, and neuroplasticity ensures that this particular circuitry within the brain gets reinforced yet again.

Mindfulness provides us with a stable platform from which we can see clearly and act wisely in the face of strong emotion. Fear, frustration or anger; joy, excitement or love; the desired emotions and the unwelcome ones all deserve our interest and curiosity if we are to live emotionally connected lives and navigate our relationships skilfully. But awareness of what is happening when a negative reaction occurs is the first essential step.

Let's imagine an alternative scenario. Your morning got off to the same start, but this time you become aware of what's happening within you much earlier.

A mindful path through anger

Walking through the house and noticing the mess you feel the wave of anger.

Somehow it registers within you that something potentially destructive could come out of this situation, so you find a chair and allow a settling to occur.

Observing the furious flow of thoughts accompanying the anger and frustration, you ground your attention in the sensations you can feel in the body—tightness around the jaw, a heavy feeling in the chest. You direct the focus of your attention to the breath, and begin a few minutes of soothing rhythm breathing.

With a kind inner voice you guide yourself through what's happening, connecting with your feelings. 'This is so disappointing. I had a plan for today, and now it's gone. It's understandable that I feel angry.'

As the intensity of the reaction subsides, instead of fuelling your anger by resentfully cleaning up the dishes from last night, you decide to go for the walk you had planned.

Walking briskly, you ground your attention by tuning in to what you see and hear. Again and again you gently direct the focus of your attention away from any images or thoughts about the mess you've left at home.

Other emotions show up, feelings of regret that the restful day you had planned now feels lost, and sadness that this situation will mean you need to find a way to speak with your partner about the disappointment.

Gradually you feel more relaxed.

So often when anger arises, there are other feelings beneath it, like sadness or longing, which remain concealed when the power of anger fuels a wave of thoughts and actions. But in making time to pause and step away from destructive reactivity, we give ourselves a chance to find ways to avoid reinforcing disconnection.

Resilient relationships are built upon the ability to see moments of potential conflict as opportunities to plan calm and assertive conversations.

Reflection

Can you recall a time when you reacted to something that happened by 'bottling up' strong negative emotion, hoping that the whole situation would just pass? Anger often arises in situations where it would be appropriate to be assertive in a considered way. In looking back now on the situation we experimented with above, where you felt let down by your partner, is there a way in which you could imagine expressing your disappointment and frustration to them which might be helpful for the relationship in the longer term? ■

Beyond life's inevitable challenges

> " The dark does not destroy the light,
> it defines it. It's our fear of the dark that
> casts our joy into the shadows. "

— Brené Brown, a professor at the University of Houston, whose research and teaching have contributed greatly to the understanding of why it is so important to face our vulnerabilities with courage and compassion

Much of the pressure behind keeping busy in life has to do with trying to distance ourselves from the difficulty of coming to terms with what it means to be human.

In reality there is really very little of what happens to us that we can control; and it can be painful to accept the fact that no matter how hard we try, we cannot completely protect those who are dear to us. The challenge to not escape into an existence of automatic pilot becomes all the more difficult when, with the flick of a switch, we can turn on our televisions and have the world news broadcast into our living room.

Vivid images of suffering and hardship, which call for our attention. How can we feel the pain of this and yet drop back into 'normal' life? For most, the solution is to develop our own 'bulletproof' armour, but we rarely notice that it is emotion and not bullets that we are trying to escape from. This sort of protection comes at a cost, a big cost.

When we try to turn away from things which haunt or frighten us, we become more generally numb to emotion; the process can't be done selectively. When we turn away from fear, longing or sadness, we are also shutting out depth in the sensations of joy, happiness and contentment.

Laura's story

Laura and Ted were a young couple pregnant with their first child. They had migrated from Scotland for Ted's work two years previously. Laura came to see me because she was concerned about a deep sadness, which seemed to come from the awareness of knowing that she would be raising her family thousands of miles away from her parents and sister back home.

Laura was a sensitive young woman. Back in Scotland she had worked as a journalist, reporting on international affairs, and her special interest was humanitarian issues and the way they played out in world politics. Since moving to Australia she had begun to write occasional articles for a national newspaper.

When Laura first saw me she already had experience with a mindfulness practice she had learned when she took part in an eight-week Mindfulness Based Stress Reduction course back in Edinburgh. She had been treated for anxiety in the past, but was strongly committed to getting through her pregnancy without taking medication if possible.

Most days Laura made time to do a body scan meditation, but although her formal practice had given her great strength in the past, she was troubled by the fact that the longing for her family and home in Scotland continued to dominate her days.

The intrusive feelings were getting in the way of Laura feeling connected to the baby she was carrying, and that added to her distress.

Almost without exception, the aspects of life which challenge or confuse us, or cause us pain, are inextricably connected to issues which are central to our experience of life and what is most meaningful to us.

During her pregnancy, far away from extended family, Laura encountered anxiety again. The way she had used her mindfulness practice up to that point seemed not to get close to touching the anguish she now felt. When we spoke in more detail about how she was using her daily meditation, it seemed to me that Laura had begun to use the time as a means of escape, a way of getting relief from the difficult feelings that gnawed away, quietly but almost continuously, at other times.

Meditation instruction is a bit like a map, or an instruction showing us how to guide the focus of our attention. Meditation is not a destination; it will disappoint us if we try to use it as a place to retreat to from life.

As I got to know Laura, together we designed a new meditation practice that was intended to connect her at least symbolically to the very aspects of her life that she could not control, and from which she did not really want to escape. Laura lived very close to a beautiful suburban beach. Each day she walked along the water's edge. We decided to use this as a place for a walking meditation.

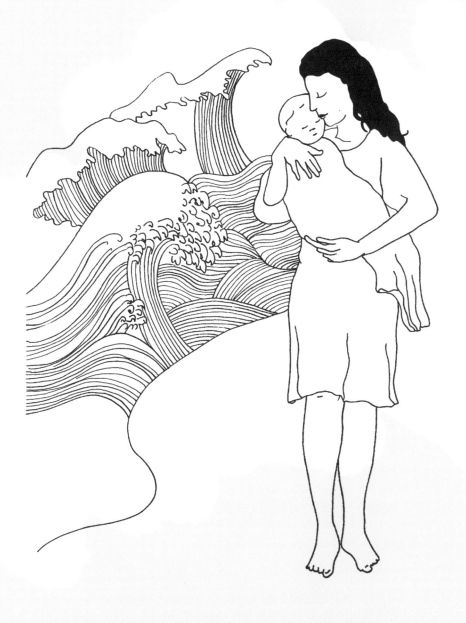

Meditation teaches us to face our fears and worries rather than retreat from them

Laura's beach meditation

As you walk towards the water's edge, allow your attention to be grounded in the sense of movement in your body.

Notice the rhythm of your steps; slow your pace just enough so that you can consciously be aware of what it feels like to have the sand shifting beneath your feet.

If it feels right, you might want to take your shoes off; allow the coolness of the sand and the occasional wave to wash over your skin. Ground yourself again and again to these sensations.

Lift your head and take in all you can see and hear—the movement of people on the shoreline; the sound of cars in the distance; and the stretch of water leading to the distant horizon. Allow your attention to stabilise in all of this activity of life.

Now, as much as is comfortable, imagine that out beyond the horizon, somewhere many miles away, is your family. See if you can hold this in your awareness; images of your parents, your sister, might come to mind. Simply hold these images lightly, while connecting still to the sense of being grounded on the earth.

Connect to any feelings in your heart, any longing or sadness, whatever arises. If at any time it feels too much, simply quicken your step, shift the focus of your attention back to the physical sensations of the sand beneath your feet, the vision of the water and the horizon.

If it's comfortable, allow yourself to feel a deep sense of connection and kindness to others, to your husband, to your family, to anyone who comes to mind—those you know and perhaps those you don't know. Just allowing a sense of belonging to a broader community, people who, just like you, are doing the best they can with their lives.

In this way Laura learned how to simply be with these very significant emotions. As she came to trust this mindfulness space she created for herself, Laura found that she could more spontaneously bring courage and wisdom to the times when she was really missing her family. Laura learned to be discerning with regard to when she allowed herself to watch confronting news items. In the months before her baby was born, she returned to her journalism with increased energy. Laura found she was able to explore the issues facing refugees and the homeless with more ease and acceptance.

This heightened awareness of the complexity of human life was a beautiful and essential part of who Laura was. Her anxiety gradually settled and in the final trimester of her pregnancy she told me that she was excited to meet her child. While this quality of sensitivity could at times lead to her feeling vulnerable, it also deeply connected her to the spirit of human existence.

Reflection

Many situations we struggle with are an inevitable part of life's journey. Laura learned how to adapt her mindfulness practice in such a way that it helped her face and simply be with her inner pain. Are there any aspects of your life which you tend to turn away from? Perhaps they bring feelings of loneliness, longing or fear? Maybe a loss from the past, or a fear for the future? Can simply holding the word 'courage' in mind provide you with a sense of inner stability from which you can allow these difficult feelings or memories to simply be? ■

Noticing reactivity

P ure, clear and uncomplicated attention, the kind of focus that allows us to simply rest in the richness of the present moment—this is what mindfulness has to offer.

Much like a crystal clear pond of water, from the space of mindfulness we can see everything that the mind offers up: happiness, sadness, judgements and fear. The shifting and largely unpredictable feast that comes with being human.

And in the same way that the surface of a pond might get choppy and rough at times, the activity in our mind can toss us around and temporarily obscure from our vision the stability that lies just beneath the surface.

But the stability is always there, just waiting for us.

Richard's story

Becoming a father changed Richard's life in ways he had never anticipated. When he was 41 years old, Richard had all but given up on the possibility of finding a partner and becoming a parent. But when he met Erin four years ago, it felt as if his personal life had finally turned around. When he first came to see me, Richard and Erin were expecting their second baby and their first child Anna was two years old.

Although Richard had come to parenting a bit later in life than most of his friends, he had not lacked confidence. He assumed quite logically that his training as a psychologist and all his years of experience working closely with people would be rich and unique preparation for family life.

In his first session with me, I noticed how intently focused Richard was upon the disappointment he felt with himself as a father. Life was hectic and especially busy since Erin left the workforce to have Anna. Richard was left with the sole responsibility of generating an income for the family, as well as doing what he could to support his wife in the challenges she experienced coping with morning sickness and parenting their energetic young toddler.

Richard felt that he wasn't handling his stress very well at all. He was most concerned about the way in which irritability and impatience were impacting upon his relationship with Anna. She was at a challenging age and was often rebellious, and it frustrated him that he lacked confidence and ease in handling her behaviour.

Anna had begun insisting that her mother put her to bed at night, refusing to allow him to read her a bedtime story. As Anna began experimenting with her first few words, Richard felt a deep sense of shame when he began hearing her say, 'No Daddy! Go away'.

When we observe how the human mind works, reactivity is the term that is used for the process by which the focus of our attention is pulled away from the present moment. Looking more carefully at the early murmurings of this experience of turning away, we usually see some sort of discomfort. Sometimes it is simply boredom.

For Richard, it was the pain of hearing his daughter's protests that woke strong reactivity within him. Reactivity contributed to his irritability and impatience. For Richard to find mindfulness helpful in this situation, he first needed to be able to recognise what was happening.

One of the most significant lessons we can learn when using mindfulness is the wisdom and effectiveness of turning towards reactivity, learning from it and grounding ourselves in the face of it.

Reactivity occurring in our relationships can be a difficult and at times painful experience. For Richard, the desire to be a good father and husband was now central to his purpose in life, and each time Anna exposed his lack of confidence and irritability by behaving just as we would expect a toddler to behave, Richard became vulnerable to reactivity.

One of the most significant lessons we can learn when using mindfulness is the wisdom and effectiveness of turning towards reactivity, learning from it and grounding ourselves in the face of it.

In his work as a psychologist, Richard had received some training in mindfulness, so the concepts were not unfamiliar to him, but he had never established a regular personal practice. With the eventual aim of using mindfulness to work more directly with reactivity in his relationship with his daughter, I asked Richard to begin a daily mindfulness of the breath practice.

We chose to refer to this as his soothing rhythm breathing, drawing from the way that Professor Paul Gilbert uses a breathing practice to cultivate strength in the emotional system of compassion. Remember, a mindfulness practice inevitably opens our eyes to all the activity going on in the stress and striving systems.

We need to be ready to turn to the compassion system, otherwise known as the connected or calm and safe system of emotion, which gives us access to the essential qualities we need in life—courage, stability, wisdom and kindness.

We can use mindfulness practice as a way of building resilience, much like we can use yoga to build strength and flexibility in our body and in our mind. In the exercise that follows I take Richard through a process called 'exposure', a basic psychological technique used to reduce reactivity.

Feel free to try this exercise, but make sure you begin with something to which you have only a small or moderate amount of reactivity, something which is not too distressing. At any time, if anxiety or another tough emotion takes over, let the exercise go, take a walk and connect to your breath and all you can see, hear and feel in the present moment.

Inviting reactivity in—an exercise

Sit comfortably on a chair with your feet flat on the floor. Allow your posture to be erect and dignified. As best you can, try to be both relaxed and alert.

Soften the muscles around your face and shoulders, and bring a soft smile to the expression on your face. This will encourage a spirit of welcome and openness to whatever images or thoughts arise.

Direct the focus of your attention gently to the sensation of the breath moving through the body, from the nose, all the way down to the abdomen. You might find it helpful to count as you breathe—to five on the in-breath, then a small pause, then to five on the out-breath. Thoughts will come and go; that's absolutely fine and to be expected. As best you can, let them go and return the focus of your awareness to the breath.

Now, for about one minute, we are going to invite into this space of mindfulness the memory of a challenging time. As best you can, bring to mind a memory of when you were struggling in your connection with someone who you are close to. It might be an experience of being with your child, your partner or perhaps someone you work with. Just allow the memory of this experience to be there; it might be a stable or fleeting image, or sounds.

What can you hear? What can you see? Can you name any emotions—perhaps fear, sadness or frustration? Can you notice any sensations in your body—perhaps a tightness or heaviness? Allow any images, feelings and thoughts that arise to just be there.

Okay, now we are going to come back to the awareness of the breath. Patiently but firmly redirect the focus of your attention back to the physical sensation of the movement of the breath. In this way we are practising a 'letting go' of thoughts and images.

Now we are going to invite in a different image. As best you can, bring to mind a memory of this special person smiling with you, the memory of a time when the two of you felt much closer, happy to be with each other. The image might be quite fleeting; that's perfectly okay. As best you can, see if you can bring awareness to any feelings or emotions. If you quickly scan through your body, are there any physical sensations you can notice?

Allow your attention to settle again with the breath. Soften into any tension you can feel in your body, and as best you can let go of any images, thoughts or body sensations. Return again to an awareness of the movement of your breath and a sense of being right here, in this moment.

When you are ready, open your eyes and bring your awareness back to the room.

In this practice we are deliberately learning how to shift from a mode of reactivity to one of calm stability, how to notice reactivity but not be swept up by it.

In day-to-day life, mindfulness invites us to notice reactivity but not to judge it or take it too seriously. Reactivity wants to be taken seriously; it's itching for a response from the thinking mind, eager to race down the nearest pathway of rumination and problem-solving.

There was no doubt in my mind that in his training as a psychologist and in his ongoing work as a therapist, Richard had developed considerable insight into his emotional life and the way previous life experience had shaped his personality. However, as we all know, we can never be totally prepared for strong emotional reactions that arise, especially when we are tired or stressed or when important relationships are strained.

One way in which we can actively use mindfulness to prepare for this is to 'invite in' to a formal practice, for a brief period of time, a troubling memory or an imagined situation that we would like to manage with more skill and wisdom. The human mind works as a powerful simulator. When we bring situations to life in an imagined way we are swept up in a flood of hormones and firing of nerve cell circuitry which affects our emotions and the type of thoughts we have, just as if the situation was happening in the present moment. Richard learned what it felt like in his body to have strong negative emotions like irritability, anger and sadness arising, and also more nourishing emotions such as happiness, joy and a sense of feeling safe. By redirecting the focus of his attention back to the movement of his breath, he was building strength in his capacity to stabilise his emotions and slow down any potentially unhelpful reactivity.

Just one word of caution—if you choose to try this exercise, it is important not to begin with a very difficult situation, it will be unhelpful if the memory causes overwhelming emotion.

Reflection

Are there any particular situations that predictably cause you to feel irritable or angry? Get to know these triggers for reactivity, but instead of allowing them to run the show, play around instead with finding stability in their midst. Try getting some distance from what is happening, or what your thoughts might be telling you, by saying quietly to yourself, 'Ahh, reactivity—I can see you'. ■

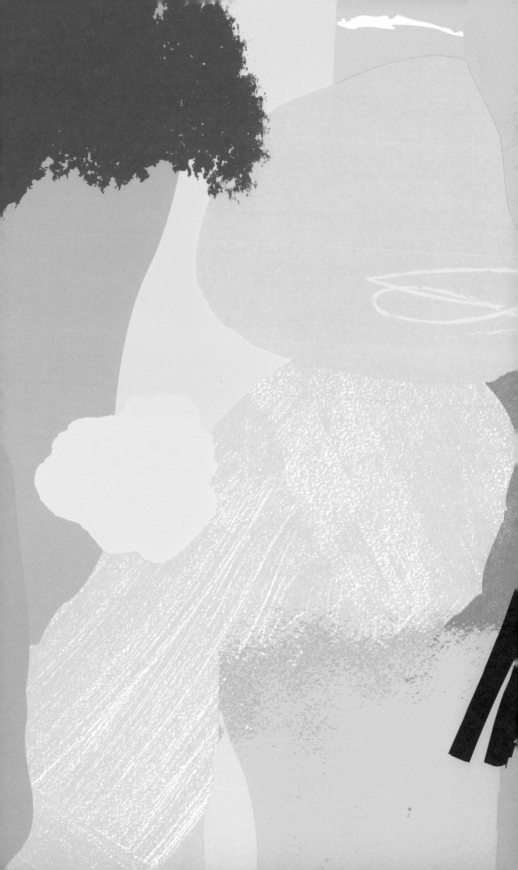

Lesson
17

Your
child's
mind

Time out, star charts, consequences—how well do they really work? Let's face it, it's easy to get confused with parenting, no matter how old the child might be. A strategy that works brilliantly with challenging behaviour one day is just as likely to fail miserably the next. So why is it that the task of raising children is not more logical and predictable?

It seems that the answer relates more to biology and the way children's brains develop than previous generations ever imagined. In humans, the process of hardwiring nerve cell connections between the part of the brain responsible for emotion (the limbic system) and the frontal lobes is not complete until the mid-twenties. This means that when the threat system fires up in a child or adolescent and they feel angry, anxious or afraid, it is much harder for them to call upon the capacities of the frontal lobes to ride the wave of the emotion and respond wisely rather than impulsively.

Tim's story

A loud crashing noise came from Tim's bedroom as he flung his homework book at the wall. 'That stupid teacher—I hate her,' he yelled.

Lucas, Tim's father, threw an angry look at his wife before racing down the passage to deal with his son. He was tired of feeling as if he was the only person actively parenting this young boy.

'How dare you throw your book and refer to your teacher like that. No iPad for a week, and I don't want to see you again this evening until your homework is done and you're ready for bed,' he roared at his son.

Tim's parents couldn't be further apart in their approach to managing the behaviour of their twelve-year-old son. Tim's mother Julie thought it was crucial to be a kind parent—she rarely raised her voice and, more often than not, when he approached his mother with a request, Tim got what he wanted.

As you might imagine, this created big problems in the family, because Lucas was convinced that his son was being spoiled. What really got Lucas mad, though, was when Tim answered his father back or didn't seem to appreciate what adults were doing for him.

Like most parents, Julie and Lucas were both motivated to do what they thought was best for their son. Lucas wanted to make sure that his son would grow up to be responsible, respectful and independent. Julie agreed with these values, but she believed their son was a sensitive child; she enjoyed seeing him happy and she felt sure that harsh discipline was not the way to bring out the best in Tim. Like in many families, Tim, Lucas and Julie are caught up in repetitive and unhelpful cycles of reacting to emotion.

If we try to understand what is going on for Tim as he hurls his book at the wall and curses his teacher, it's reasonable to assume that his amygdala is firing strongly and the level of stress hormone cortisol will be high. In fact, the stress response probably started well before the dramatic book launch. Struggling to make sense of his homework, as emotion in his limbic system began to dominate the way his brain was working, Tim's capacity to concentrate, pay attention and problem solve would have been deteriorating rapidly. We can guess that in the grip of these overwhelming emotions Tim probably felt alone, that his teacher didn't care about him and that he was never going to be able to understand the difficult maths project.

When his father storms into his room with a list of consequences, how helpful do you think that might be? Is it likely that Tim will say, 'Sorry, Dad, I didn't mean to lose it', and get on with his homework in a more orderly way? When parents respond in ways that increase a child's level of distress by yelling, smacking or isolating them from others, activity within the amygdala increases.

In this case, neuroplasticity will ensure that Tim's memory of this evening will be laid down together with many painful emotions. The result of this is likely to be that the next time he struggles with maths, it is more likely that Tim will feel unsettled or even anxious, which in turn will affect his ability to concentrate and focus, setting the scene for another potential meltdown.

So, if the aim is to help Tim learn how to get to the other side of a distressing emotional wave of helplessness and anger without losing it, how else might Lucas and Julie respond? To work this out, it will be helpful to begin by exploring what is currently understood about the emotional wellbeing of children.

Perhaps not surprisingly, long-term research suggests that children who are able to regulate their emotions are more likely to be confident in their relationships, optimistic and resilient in their moods and do well academically. These skills of understanding and regulating emotions are often referred to as emotional intelligence.

The highly respected child parenting program Circle of Security suggests the most effective way of teaching emotional intelligence to children is to help them tolerate, label and make sense of their emotions. They call this being with the emotions of our children. This method regards discipline as essential too, but the aim should always be to teach children rather than punish them.

But how might this translate into strategies for parenting?

Circle of Security teaches parents to pause before responding when

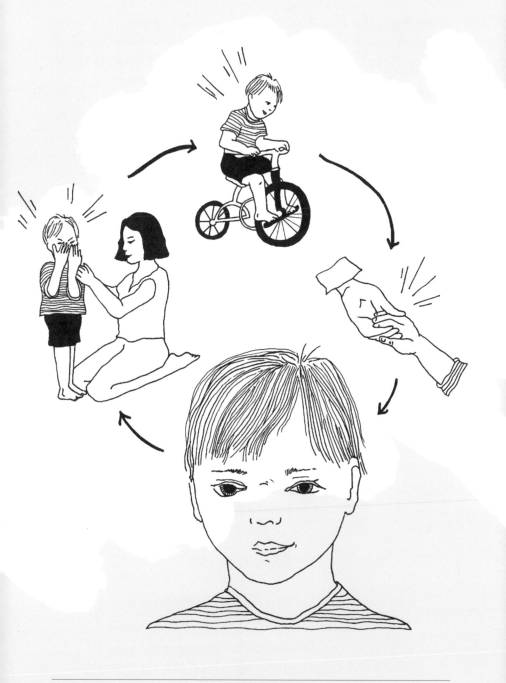

Circle of Security

when their child is distressed. Like in any other relationship, strong emotions inevitably and automatically (via the activity of mirror neurones) trigger similar emotions in those around them. When we remember to pause, we give ourselves the opportunity to check in, making sure that we are not about to add more negativity to an already difficult situation.

Long-term research suggests that children who are able to regulate their emotions are more likely to be confident in their relationships, optimistic and resilient in their moods and do well academically.

The Circle of Security program has a helpful way of describing what we need to aim for: no matter what is happening, whether we think the behaviour is deliberate or not, always aim to be *bigger, stronger, wiser and kind.* In his books on parenting (see the Resources section) child psychiatrist Dr Dan Siegel echoes this perspective. He cautions us to remember that it is precisely when our children are out of control that they need us the most. Experts in the area of children's emotional wellbeing agree that discipline is essential, but it will be more likely to have the desired effect when it is logical and delivered with warmth and respect.

One way to understand this is to imagine that as a parent your responsibility is to provide the link between your child's amygdala and their frontal lobes. So let's imagine how things might have turned out if Lucas and Julie had been able to ride the waves of their own quite logical emotions of anger and fear, and responded to Tim's behaviour from this *bigger, stronger, wiser and kind* position.

Dad's repair

Hearing the loud noise from Tim's room, Lucas looks at his wife and says quietly, 'He's having a rough time again.'

Heading for Tim's bedroom, Lucas drops into a more mindful space and does what he can to settle his own emotions. He walks slowly, noticing and letting go of tension being held in the muscles of his face and shoulders while he grounds his attention so his thoughts don't race away.

He reminds himself that while he is unhappy with Tim's explosive behaviour, his son has been struggling with maths, and the best thing he can do at this moment is try to help his son see things more clearly.

The first thing that Tim notices is that his father is calm. Maybe it's safe to let down his guard.

Sitting down beside Tim, Lucas puts a hand on his son's knee and says kindly, 'Hey, it's okay, I'm here. It sounds like you're feeling pretty angry. Do you feel up to talking about it?'

With that, there is a flood of tears. After a minute or so Tim is calmer, and he says to his dad, 'I hate it; I just don't get this maths. My teacher is useless.'

'That's really tough,' says Lucas. 'I can remember what it was like to not understand what's going on in class. What say we take a break, do you feel like a walk? We can come back to this later. Perhaps I might be able to make sense of it with you.'

There were a few steps that Lucas followed here. He not only helped Tim feel that his emotions made sense, but, by sharing his own memories from school, helped Tim feel that he was not alone. Labelling emotion has been shown to reduce activity in the amygdala—Dr Dan Siegel calls this step 'name it to tame it'. Physical activity can really help balance emotion—and not just for children.

Reflection

Are there any familiar traps that you fall into when it comes to disciplining your child? Can you recognise what emotions take over when you react to your child's behaviour in a way that you later regret? ■

The science of positivity and optimism

The seeds of happiness and optimism, just like compassion and wisdom, are present in all of us. Just like their more pessimistic cousins, the nerve cell circuitry of positive emotions and thinking patterns obey the same principles of neuroplasticity.

In our search for happiness, most of us make the mistake of waiting for something specific to happen—another holiday, a different job or better behaviour from a child. But sooner or later most of us come to understand that this 'outsourcing' of happiness is a risky business. Researchers call it the 'hedonic treadmill'. Hardwired into the striving and pleasure-seeking system of emotion, getting the things we desire can give us an intoxicating rush of positive feelings.

In fact, similar changes occur in the body's internal chemistry with the use of addictive substances like cocaine and amphetamine, which is why we can get 'addicted' to shopping or fad diets or gambling. The biochemistry of this pleasure circuitry activates quickly but falls even more rapidly, taking with it our mood.

Lisa's journey through depression

Lisa had taken antidepressant medication as treatment for depression for many years. She had managed to avoid postnatal depression after the births of each of her three children and attributed her new-found emotional resilience to participating in a course of Mindfulness Based Cognitive Therapy during her first pregnancy.

The course taught her how to build steadiness in her mind and observe the activity of her thoughts while resisting any pull to engage in a debate with them. Then, as she learned how to bring this capacity to be focused in the moment to her parenting, she found that she could connect more deeply in the interactions she had with her children.

But when Lisa came to see me, she explained that although her life had great meaning and she no longer felt particularly frightened of depression, she found great difficulty feeling positive and hopeful about the world her children were growing up in. How would she feel if one of her children became depressed like she had been? How could she protect them from experiences which might cause them to suffer?

Positive emotions such as joy and happiness are fragile and are no match for the strength of negative emotions which dominate our thoughts when our inner threat system gets activated.

Apart from the fact that we get more pleasure from life when happiness and joy grace our day, there are other important reasons why positive emotions are worthy of our attention. The work of two well-respected researchers into human emotion, Professor Barbara Fredrickson and Professor Richard Davidson, has demonstrated how positive emotions radically change the way our brains operate, and how with regular practice positivity alters the physical structure of our brains. Rather than positive emotions being the result of success in life, it seems that the reverse is actually the case—success in work life and relationships comes more readily to those who are able to draw upon positive emotions such as gratitude, hope, pride and love.

Professor Fredrickson's research shows that positivity does not follow 'linear' dynamics. In other words, the more often we choose to take in the positive, the more likely it will be that positive meaning will come spontaneously from experiences which might otherwise have felt unremarkable. Research measuring emotional resilience in survivors of trauma such as the 9/11 terrorist attacks in the United States, showed that people who managed to connect with others rather than retreat, to focus on what felt precious rather than what was frightening did substantially better in their lives as the years went on.

When the function of the brain is observed, it appears that positivity opens up awareness of what is happening around us, while negative emotions like irritability, pessimism and doubt tend to close awareness down. Under the influence of negative emotions it can feel as if we have tunnel vision.

While Lisa's concerns about her mood were important, we needed to move beyond any expectation that treating her depression was on its own going to spontaneously lead to greater happiness. Together we found ways to build upon Lisa's regular mindfulness practice by using imagery and learning how to bring more focused attention to aspects of her life that tended to pass by unnoticed.

Lisa's positivity exercises

Lisa began her ten-minute morning practice while lying quietly in bed, first settling her mind by focusing for a couple of minutes on the sensations of her in-breath and out-breath at the tip of her nose. She then brought to mind memories of enjoyable experiences. One of her favourites was a recent family holiday at the beach. As best she could Lisa brought to life images of her children jumping over waves, shrieking with delight, and her partner holding her hand as they watched, waves washing over their toes. Focusing on what she could see, hear and feel, each day she practised she found these rich memories came to life more vividly.

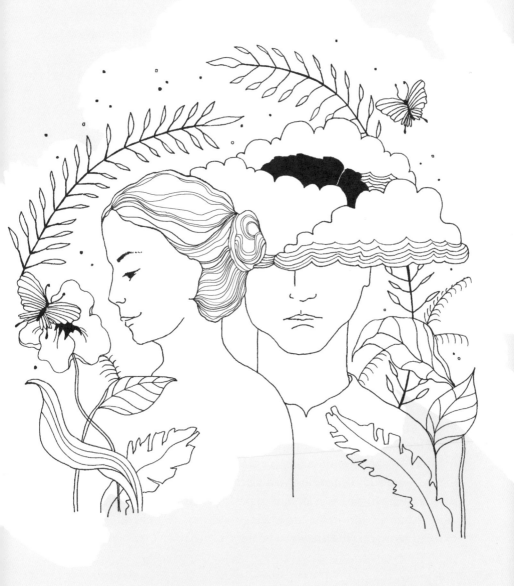

Positivity opens our awareness; negativity shuts it down

At the end of each day Lisa made time for another brief practice. Beginning with some relaxing yoga stretches, she then sat quietly and brought to her mind what had gone well that day. Surprisingly, with practice she found it increasingly less difficult to find things to feel glad about—the warm greeting of the barista who made her morning coffee, or the kind word of one of her colleagues who always asked after Lisa's family. Lisa brought these memories to life as vividly as she could, feeling the warmth of the emotions as connected to the way they felt in her body.

Over the next few weeks as her practice became more solid and rich, Lisa found that through the day she was spontaneously noticing enjoyable experiences more often. It felt so nourishing that she decided to find ways to weave this focus upon positive experiences into her interactions with her partner and children. Instead of allowing dinnertime to be simply a time of distracted interactions, Lisa tried to find ways in which she could support family conversations, encouraging more focus on discussions that arose.

You might notice that the experiences Lisa chose to play back and treasure involved times she had spent with other people. One common finding of research into a more authentic happiness is that it tends to be linked to having close relationships with others.

One word of caution—if you give the following exercise a go, keep in mind that positive thoughts are fragile; it's very easy for the rational mind to quickly dismantle the delicacy of the good feelings. We are simply trying to weave in strands of positivity through the day, trying to gently shift the inevitable underlying tendency we were all born with, to focus more on what needs to be done or what isn't quite right.

Reflection

Turning towards the positive aspects of our experiences takes practice and patience. What we choose to work with can be of less importance than the fact that we have simply made a choice to incline the mind towards the value of an experience in a more open or optimistic way. Is it possible to find a way to feel more positive about a mundane task, such as the routine grocery shopping or driving your car to complete some errands? In even considering this, can you notice the 'thinking mind' commenting with scepticism or negativity? ■

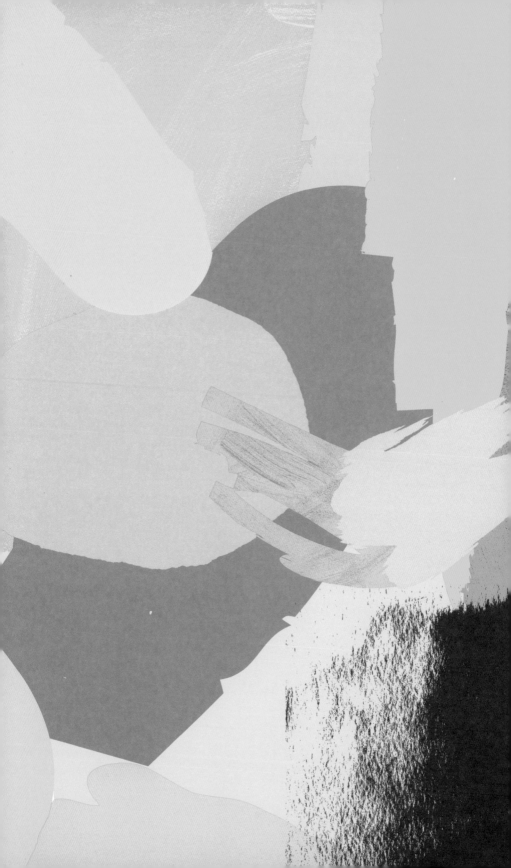

Lesson 19

Meaning making

The human mind is the ultimate meaning-making machine. In case you hadn't noticed it, our mind working quietly in the background provides a constant commentary on our lives. It seems to never tire of going over and over what is already history or working away on scenarios of what might happen, or might not, sometime in the future.

Mostly we trust our minds, blissfully unaware of the biases hardwired into the nerve cell pathways in our brains, the most significant of which has us more sensitively tuned into what might go wrong, or what we are afraid of, rather than what might be going well.

Emma's story

Emma was three months into her second pregnancy when she first came to see me. Her initial excitement had all but gone as she struggled to cope with tiredness and low mood. Her two-year-old son Billy had picked up on some of this and had become clingy and unsettled. Emma spent most of the first session with me in tears. 'I'm just not connecting with this baby,' she told me.

Emma was working full time and her mother cared for Billy when she worked. Mostly the arrangement worked well, but her mother was an anxious woman, and most days when Emma picked Billy up, her mother seemed determined to share with her daughter all the worries she had about her grandson. 'He's very picky with his food, Emma; you should take him to the doctor, I don't think he's getting enough to eat.' Or 'He's not speaking any words yet—don't you think that by this age he should be saying more?'

The well-intentioned words of her mother planted powerful seeds of worry and doubt in Emma's mind, and well beneath her conscious awareness, a process of trying to make meaning of what had been said had begun. Why was Billy's speech slow in developing? Were his temper outbursts happening because she was working and not more hands on with his care? Was her mother really trying to tell her that she was neglecting her son? If she couldn't connect to this second baby she was carrying, what did that say about how she was going to manage with two children?

She found herself dreading these interactions and noticed that she was constantly observing Billy, trying to work out what was really going on.

Emma was experiencing firsthand how, under the influence of emotions like fear and anxiety, our minds become selective in what they pay attention to. A process of making meaning of experience takes hold and so for Emma, whenever Billy refused to eat or was difficult to settle, this seemed to be more evidence in support of her mother's concerns.

This was a great example of neuroplasticity at work. As we know, 'Nerve cells that fire together wire together'. In Emma's case, this meant that the more often she got caught up with worries about bonding with her baby or being a good mother to Billy, the more likely it was that these thoughts would return with increasing strength.

Mindfulness works best when our times of formal practice are complemented by a process of weaving the skills into the more challenging areas of our life. For Emma the experiences which troubled her most were the conversations she had with her mother about Billy, times when Billy was tired and unhappy and the occasions when she began to think about her pregnancy, comparing it to how excited she had been when she carried Billy. These were the specific situations where it would be helpful if Emma could find a way to access a process of mindfulness, and disconnect from her internal 'rumour mill'.

Emma was highly motivated to learn mindfulness. She booked into a Mindfulness Based Stress Reduction Course, but that didn't begin for a few weeks, so we decided to make a start together. In order to begin the day with a practice, Emma set her morning alarm a little earlier and her husband took care of Billy, giving her uninterrupted time for one formal practice each day.

Emma's mindfulness practice

For her first week of practice, Emma followed a guided body scan meditation. At the end of that week, I suggested that she lead herself through the practice, without using the audio guide. Beginning at her feet she patiently redirected the focus of her attention slowly and systematically up through her body. As I expected, Emma found it challenging, but she remembered my reassurance that there was no such thing as an unsuccessful meditation. Each time she noticed that her mind had drifted away and managed to redirect the focus of her attention to sensations in her body, she had succeeded!

At our next catch up, in addition to her daily body scan, I asked Emma to find a couple of minutes twice during each day to 'drop into' mindfulness less formally. I suggested she set an alarm on her phone to remind her to pause and direct the focus of her attention to ten slow steady breaths. We decided that when she did this she would also put a simple label on any emotion she could detect ('worried', 'tense', 'weary'), followed by gently redirecting the focus of her attention to what was actually happening in the present moment.

Over the next few weeks Emma became more sensitively tuned in to times when her mind was wandering. She found that labelling her emotions not only helped her to settle, but also to see how close the connection was between her feelings and thoughts. Being more aware of when she felt tense or worried meant that she picked up earlier any tendency to worry about Billy.

As she progressed, we used one of our sessions together to experiment with ways Emma could interact with her mother more skilfully. We then rehearsed an interaction, and I played her mother, voicing the concerns about Billy that Emma had already heard many times before. I suggested to Emma that when she heard me speak, imaging that I was her mother, she might simply listen carefully, note any reactions going on within, such as thoughts or body sensations, or even an urge to get up and leave, but instead of getting caught up with the reaction, as best she could she would try to simply reconnect with the physical sensations of her breath moving in and out of her body.

After allowing for a few minutes of connection to the movement of her breath, I then asked Emma to consider whether it might be possible to respond to her mother in a different way.

With a renewed confidence Emma replied, 'I really appreciate all your help with Billy, Mum. I know you have concerns and I do take them seriously. I'll keep a close eye on him, but I'm pretty sure we're on the right track.'

In this practice, Emma had used her imagination to bring to life a memory of an interaction with her mother and, as expected, her mind began to work as a powerful simulator. Just imagining the concerned voice of her mother was enough to lead to a surge of worried thoughts, and a physical sensation of tightness in her body.

Reflection

Can you think of a situation that feels loaded for you, in which the stories you hold about the situation tend to focus too much on a limited perspective? Is it possible to hold an image of this situation in your mind, while at the same time simply bringing a more clear awareness of the thoughts and worries that arise? In working with difficult situations with mindfulness, the intention is to practise letting go of any desire to engage in a debate with our thoughts. We notice that worrying thoughts are present, but patiently redirect the focus of our attention to an awareness of the present moment. In such an exercise, our goal would not be to solve a problem, or manipulate the way in which we are interpreting what is going on, but simply to be with the experience and observe the reaction that is happening. Occasionally, however, as occurred in this exercise with Emma, a wiser way of understanding the difficulty might spontaneously come to us. ■

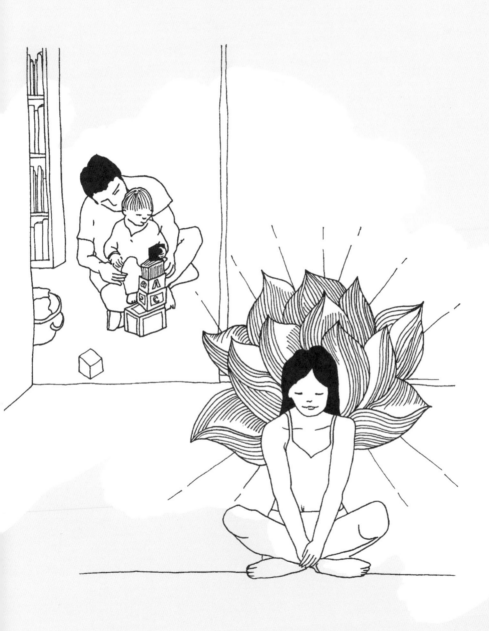

Making space in a busy life for mindfulness

Lesson
20

Equanimity

Equanimity—it's a word barely used in modern society, but even holding the concept in our minds can help provide us with a roadmap to a different place when what is going on around us feels tough. A place where we can simply stand and observe. Equanimity is perhaps best regarded as a process of non-reactivity. Rather than denying what is difficult, we learn to see things as they really are, and resist being caught up by the reactivity in our minds. Neither cold nor rigid, equanimity is infused with wisdom and kindness.

Amelia's story

Amelia was halfway through her third pregnancy. The baby she was carrying felt very large; her back gave her pain and her sleep was interrupted. Her five-year-old daughter and two-year-old son were picking up on their mother's tiredness and irritability and had become cranky and unsettled.

When she came to see me, Amelia described an inner restlessness which gripped her mind, pulling her down into a quagmire of negative thoughts. The unsettled behaviour of her young children was robbing her of confidence in her mothering, and her obstetrician had become concerned that she might be developing signs of depression.

Amelia was keen to learn skills of mindfulness, but the prospect of being left alone in a meditation with the activity of her mind felt impossibly tough. So, instead, I suggested that Amelia begin working with a skilled yoga teacher, providing her mind with the somewhat less difficult task of working with the way tension was held in her body.

Her daily practices were neither comfortable nor easy. Again and again Amelia used movement and slow, steady breathing to reach deep into the tightness and resistance that had developed in her body. Gradually, after each practice Amelia became aware of a feeling of inner quietness. She had managed to find a way to inhabit her body, and find a solid place within from which she could observe the activity of her mind without getting hauled into reactivity.

After two weeks of daily practice, Amelia's inner restlessness had begun to settle and she was more tuned in to the messages her body was giving her. During the day she was able to tell when she was ready to tackle routine tasks, but also notice when she needed to put her feet up and rest.

Yoga is a very strong practice of mindfulness. It teaches a particular quality of attention, one which is strong while also being sensitive, kind and discerning. I asked Amelia to observe the inner process of her yoga practice, the way she could direct the focus of her attention away from the activity of her mind, into the movement of her breath and the sensations in her body.

As the weeks passed, we looked for ways in which the strengths Amelia was building could be taken beyond the times of her formal practice, and

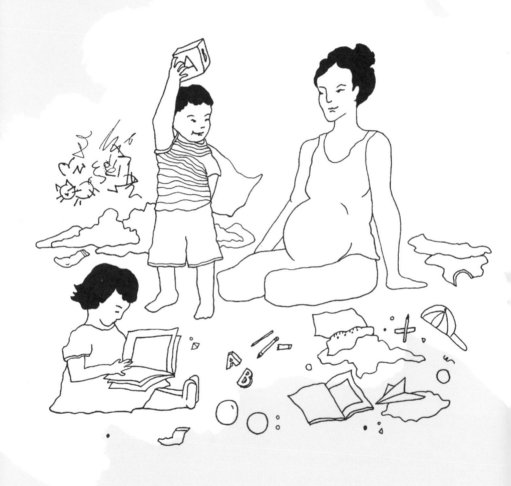

Practising equanimity is possible in everyday situations

applied more broadly to daily life. The obvious place to begin was in the time she spent with her children and the times when pain in her body threatened to pull her mind into a reaction of worry and confusion. These challenges became the beginning of Amelia's informal practice.

At times of the day when her children were tired and unsettled and her own irritability was rising, instead of relying upon directing them with her words, Amelia came to see the value in simply being with them. Seating herself comfortably, Amelia grounded her attention in body sensations, and allowed her gaze to rest on the activity of her children. Noticing the way tension was held in her body, Amelia deepened and slowed the rhythm of her breathing and allowed it to penetrate deeply into any tightness. She adjusted her posture so that she was sitting more upright, softening the expression on her face so that instead of reacting to their mother's frown, the children felt drawn to be close to her.

66

I've lived through some terrible things in my life,
some of which actually happened.

99

– *Mark Twain*

Finding equanimity

As her pregnancy progressed into the third trimester, Amelia encountered a complication which meant that she had to spend much of the day resting in bed in order to reduce the chance of a premature delivery.

Despite the help of everyone who rallied around, Amelia found it very difficult to rest. Our next session together was spent with Amelia in tears much of the time. The sense of calm and stability she had found in previous months had vanished.

'My life's been turned upside down. My mind just races ahead all the time imagining how difficult it's going to be to get Harriet and Sam back into a routine and at the same time manage a new baby. I just don't think I can do it!'

All of these painful feelings and thoughts needed space to be heard. It was not going to be helpful for me to rush in and try to help Amelia find a practical solution to her problems. She needed to feel that her distress was understandable and that I was concerned for her, but at the same time I wanted to give her the opportunity to allow the strong wave of emotions to settle and to see what emerged. So, watching her carefully, I allowed a silence to settle in the room.

'Can you put a name to some of these emotions you are feeling Amelia?'

After a minute or two she slowly replied, 'Fear, worry and I suppose if I'm really honest—anger too.'

As we gently explored what was going on beneath the fear and panic, what emerged was Amelia's awareness of the difficulty she encountered with Simon whenever she tried to talk to him about what help she might be able to get in managing the care of the children. 'Everyone tells me I am so lucky to have a husband like Simon. But it's not so great. He's been putting an effort in over the last two weeks, but I think that's just because he knows he has no choice. Work comes first in his world, and Fridays are always dinner out with the boys. Whenever I try and talk to him about the extra help I'm going to need with a new baby, it's usually when I'm fed up and we both just get angry.'

Hormonal changes of the third trimester and the worry about her pregnancy were feeding in to the activation of Amelia's threat system. Under its influence, the memories that were available to her related only to times when she had encountered difficulty with Simon's behaviour, but I knew her well enough to know that under different circumstances she had the ability to be quite skilful in her marriage. Equanimity in this situation would mean that Amelia could allow difficult emotions to arise and pass through her without becoming caught up in them, unintentionally reinforcing repetitive cycles of negativity and doubt.

Confined to her bed for many hours a day, she was no longer able to practise yoga so we modified Amelia's mindfulness practice. Once a day, when her parents took the children out of the house for a walk, she would perform a twenty-minute body scan. Whenever she felt her baby move or became aware of pain or discomfort, I suggested she practise redirecting the focus of her attention to those sensations until they changed or passed. Whatever thoughts or worries might be present, she was to try and patiently return the focus of her attention to bodily sensations; this was a way of hardwiring equanimity, or non-reactivity, to potentially distressing feelings and thoughts.

We could also try using a mindfulness practice to activate the safe and connected system of emotion. I asked Amelia if she could recall a peaceful and happy time she had experienced with her family, and she told me about a holiday they had taken at a beachside resort. Amelia had enjoyed swimming while hearing Simon and the children laughing and playing in the shallows. So, before Simon arrived home each day, Amelia took time for another brief meditation, where she brought to life images and memories of what it felt like to be swimming in the warm water, listening to her family and feeling joyful. From this calmer emotional state Amelia managed to bring a more grounded and wise approach to conversations with Simon about the additional help needed when the baby arrived. She found he listened when she spoke slowly and quietly, simply making suggestions for him to think further about.

Reflection

Becoming familiar with how it feels to have an inner restlessness can be a useful way of building insight into our 'habits' of reactivity. Consider your daily routine; can you predict which activities might cause inner restlessness, boredom or frustration? Is it possible to pay careful attention to these moments of discomfort, connect more deeply to the sensations in your body, and in this way perhaps observe the wave of reactivity come, then go? ■

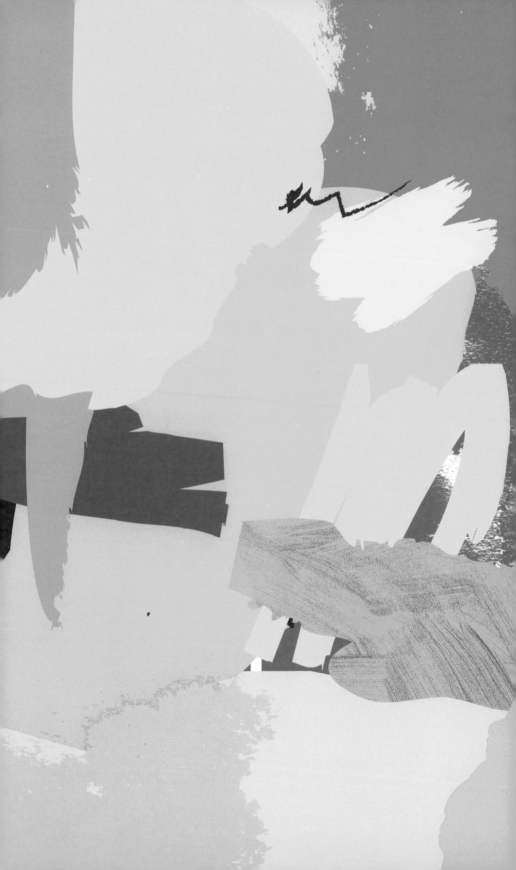

Lesson
21

Gratitude

How easy is it to take almost everything for granted? Probably much easier than it was a few decades ago, before the age of credit cards and technology enabled us to have such ready access to so many things. But has this made us happier? According to decades of study on flourishing, there is actually no evidence to suggest that gathering possessions or even achieving longed-for goals brings any lasting happiness. So where does that leave us, if we dare to accept that perhaps all of our striving may not lead to the enduring happiness that we hope for?

There is another, more hopeful, way to look at our experience of life. Research in the field of positive psychology suggests that learning how to bring emotions such as hope and gratitude into our lives on a regular basis is not only linked to lower levels of depression, but to improved physical health and more robust relationships.

So how might we begin?

Working skilfully with emotion is much like using mindfulness: we need to be patient and we need to persist. In the training of mindfulness, it is suggested we think of the skills we are developing as a way of planting seeds. These seeds will eventually grow and bear fruit, and the more seeds you plant the more lush the growth. Finding ways to cultivate gratitude is a great example of planting precious seeds, patiently noticing what would ordinarily be taken for granted, and in that moment, changing the emotional landscape of the day.

The late professor of psychology at the University of Michigan Chris Peterson and his colleagues devised a simple exercise in gratitude that was associated with increased happiness and decreased depression for up to six months of follow-up.

You might want to try it. As with many exercises in positivity, it can be interesting to simply note how the thinking mind can get in the way with an analysis or judgement of what is happening. If you choose to give the following technique a go, be patient, and try to engage in an open and curious way.

Three good things

For one week, at the end of each day, write down three things which went well during that day. These things can be quite simple and ordinarily unremarkable, or they might be more significant.

The last step is to answer: 'Why did this good thing happen?'

The researchers found that naming three good things worked better than naming ten, and doing the exercise before bed worked better than in the morning. Improved mood for up to six months was found in participants who had been asked to complete the exercise for only one week.

This is not an isolated research finding. It seems that practising gratitude is associated not only with reduced depression and increased happiness, but also better physical health. But we need to be careful in 'prescribing' gratitude, because many people who are stressed or feeling down are already asking themselves what the justification is for their unhappiness. Gratitude is not a familiar emotion in many parts of Western society, and if not done with care, bringing attention to this

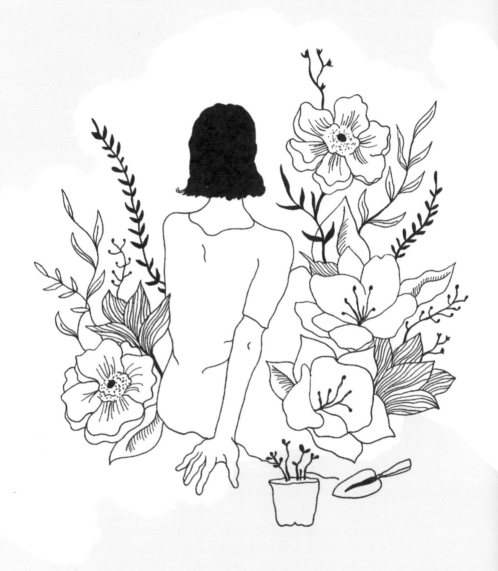

Cultivating gratitude is like planting seeds that grow and bear fruit

can really backfire, increasing self-criticism rather than helping people engage in life with more passion.

So let's see how gratitude can be a positive emotion that can make a real difference in the treatment of depression and grief.

Angela had been seeing me for about a year when we decided to take a new direction in our work together. Since separating from her husband eighteen months earlier, Angela had found it easier to cope by keeping herself busy, working and setting up a new home for herself and her three-year-old daughter Ailsa. She had initially come to see me with symptoms of depression after her husband Lucas left their marriage. A challenging part of Angela's recovery was coming to terms with the shock of losing her relationship, and she was well aware that she still held on to quite a bit of resentment.

Even though she struggled to practise regularly, training in mindfulness had helped to lift Angela's mood, restore her concentration and improve her ability to get a good night's sleep. But her irritability remained high and there were two unavoidable aspects to her life which she found particularly provocative.

Angela worked in a friendly office environment, but a significant part of her duties involved handling customer complaints on the telephone. By the end of most days she was feeling fed up and annoyed from hearing the complaints of one dissatisfied person after another. She left work feeling tense and unhappy, and she could tell that little Ailsa could sense her irritable mood when she picked her up from crèche.

Even more difficult for her, though, was the regular contact she had with Lucas and his new partner Jenny. They lived in a beautiful new house, and Ailsa had a bedroom which she shared with one of Jenny's children. When Angela dropped Ailsa off every second weekend, it was hard for her to contain her emotions. Even though she could sense that Jenny was quite nice, and was making a real effort to be polite, Angela inevitably came away feeling a horrible mix of anger and sadness.

Ailsa always seemed so happy to head off to her new home with her father and his new family, that Angela was left wondering how she was really doing in her role as a mother. I wanted to see if we could enrich Angela's mindfulness practice, by helping her find ways to engage more deeply with the aspects of life which could be nourishing for her.

We decided to focus initially on the challenging time Angela had when Ailsa was with her father. Alone in her small apartment she was familiar with many emotions, but gratitude was not one of them.

Angela's journey with gratitude

Angela woke the following Saturday morning to the quietness of her apartment. Thinking about how she might waken feelings of gratitude left her feeling sad. Wisely she decided not to rush out of bed as she tended to do. Busyness was her loyal companion on these weekends without her daughter. Instead she allowed herself to relax and began a gentle body scan meditation.

Her mind was already inclined to the task of bringing awareness to gratitude, so whenever she noticed that her mind had wandered, she said quietly to herself, 'Thank you, mind, for keeping me on track.'

After the 30-minute practice, her body felt more rested and peaceful, so she slowly got herself dressed and went through to the kitchen to make breakfast. Sitting on her balcony overlooking the local park while she ate her cereal, Angela allowed her gaze to rest on the soft green colours of the trees and grass. The sound of children playing drew her attention and she watched as parents chatted with each other and joined in with the children throwing balls and pushing swings.

A strong wave of sadness rushed over her, and this time she allowed tears to flow. It wasn't often she had the courage to cry.

After the sadness subsided, Angela returned her attention to watching the families in the park. This was her community now; she felt a sense of connection with the parents, people she had never met, and gratitude came to her and she thanked them for bringing the sounds of life to her day.

Angela later explained how that day in her apartment felt like an immersion in a different type of mindfulness. Instead of tending to her usual chores, without planning it, she ended up spending the whole day at home. She rested and she explored. She held old family photos and she allowed time to consider how precious it had been to get the support of her sister and brother through those dark months. She remembered her mother's kindness and encouragement. Gratefulness grew.

Over the next few months I witnessed a transformation in Angela. It was as if finding her way to gratitude and making time on that one precious day to allow sadness and regret to meet gratitude opened a new dimension in her ability to be mindfully present to life just as it was. Angela began to really value the company of her work colleagues, seeing them as bringing positive energy to a workplace that might otherwise feel quite bleak. As she engaged more deeply with her practice of mindfulness, energised by a spirit of gratitude, Angela began to accept that her marriage was over. Courage grew, and she allowed herself to be curious about this new woman in her daughter's life, and the pain she experienced when she dropped her daughter off diminished.

66

This is a wonderful day. I've never seen this one before.

99

— *Maya Angelou, American poet and civil rights activist*

Reflection

Try making space for gratitude in your life. Don't try to force it, be gentle and allow it to emerge quietly. But like most positive emotions, remember it will be fragile. Try to challenge or justify it, and very likely it will simply disappear. ■

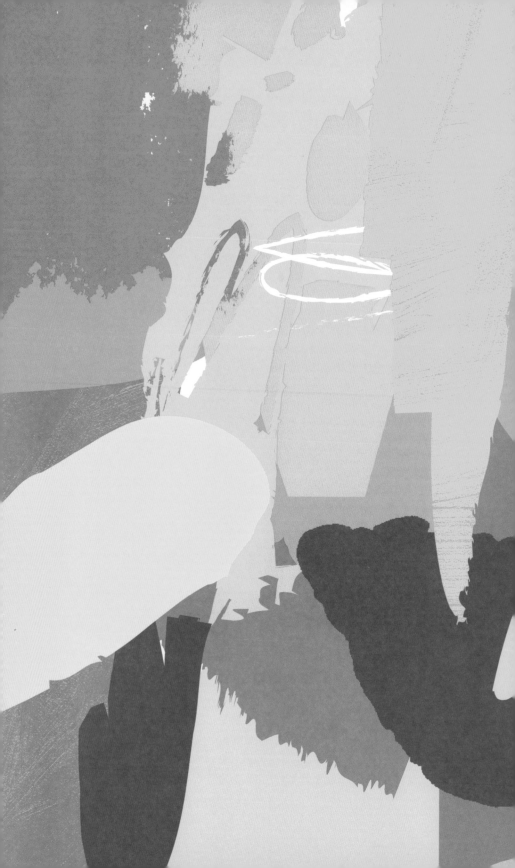

Lesson
22

Compassion

" We think that the point is to pass the test or overcome the problem, but the truth is that things don't really get solved. They come together and they fall apart. Then they come together again and fall apart again. It's just like that. The healing comes from letting there be room for all of this to happen: room for grief, for relief, for misery, for joy. "

— *Pema Chödrön, Buddhist nun, author and teacher*

As humans we are unique in our capacity for self-criticism. While we are able to accomplish amazing and wonderful things, there are no other animals that set about judging and criticising themselves, or putting themselves down, like we do. It is becoming clear that evolution has shaped the human brain in such a way that it is exquisitely sensitive and vulnerable to emotions like shame, fear and anger.

Investigating this further, it is becoming clear that self-compassion is one of the most powerful ways to bring about changes in brain architecture and function which lead to emotional resilience.

66

The way we are is not our fault. Compassion is one of the most important declarations of strength and courage known to humanity.

99

— *Paul Gilbert, Professor of Clinical Psychology,* The Huffington Post

By simply putting on the television to watch the news we are reminded of humanitarian disasters, crime and suffering that are happening on our doorsteps. How do we manage to feel calm, and to savour and cherish what we have, what feels precious, with an awareness that at the same time and perhaps not far away someone else is suffering? Knowing that perhaps tomorrow that might be us, or someone we deeply care about.

Remember the rules of neuroplasticity? 'Nerve cells that fire together wire together'—our vulnerability to distressing and potentially destructive emotions depends upon how often they are used. The more often we 'practise' fear, anger, irritability or worry, the stronger these emotions become.

As mindfulness training programs are evolving, it is becoming clear just how important it is to consider how we might strengthen the nerve cell circuitry which allows us to connect with others at times when we are in the grip of negative emotions. In my clinical practice I have found that one of the most valuable aspects of learning mindfulness in a group-based setting is receiving the support of a teacher who recognises how tough turning the attention inward can be in the face of uncomfortable thoughts or emotions; teaching self-compassion as a way of meeting inevitable hardship.

Becoming a mother

Sophia held her young daughter close to her. As baby Mia cried and squirmed, tears streamed down Sophia's cheeks.

As a first-time mother, Sophia felt completely unprepared for how life had changed. At the age of 41 she felt lost in a sleep-deprived fog, and her referral to me by her local doctor occurred after Sophia had broken down in tears in front of the small group of women in her local mothers' group.

Before leaving work to have her daughter, Sophia was a senior lawyer, running a busy private practice and volunteering at a local legal aid service. Her work had been hard but rewarding, and she had enjoyed the feeling that she was making a contribution to the lives of others who were less fortunate.

Sophia had married Matthew only one year earlier, and remembered feeling a sense of relief when she was swept off her feet in the heady first few months of their romance. At a time when she was beginning to think that she might be spending the rest of her life as a lonely career woman, Matt had come into her life with an offer of security, and a strong desire to have children.

It was not easy for Sophia to speak about her distress. She had accepted her doctor's recommendation to see me, but had never before spoken about her personal life with a stranger. I thought we might begin with what sense she was making of her experience of becoming overwhelmed in front of the other mothers.

'I don't fit in. They all look so happy. They chat away to each other about what their babies are doing, and holidays they've got planned, and I feel I've got nothing to say. It's obvious that they're finding it all so easy, and all I can think of is what is wrong with me? The other day, when one woman looked at me and asked how I was enjoying Mia, I just froze. Then I cried. No one said anything, I think they were shocked.'

Allowing a quiet pause to make space for the pain I could feel in the words she had spoken, I wondered whether it was going to be possible for Sophia to open up more to what was really going on inside.

'Well, you're the doctor, what have you got to fix this? Is there a tablet for it? A tablet that will make me a good mother?'

It was at this point that I knew we had hit gold. Somehow Sophia had found the courage to allow deep and painful feelings to emerge and be shared.

Parenting would have to be one of the most challenging jobs of all. When else in life do we take on the responsibility for the very survival and happiness of another human being? No doubt Sophia's experience in her work suggested that she already had many of the qualities that should help her feel confident as a mother—wisdom, empathy and maturity. But here she was, this intelligent and sensitive person, trapped in overwhelming feelings of inadequacy and unworthiness.

We might have strong circuitry for self-criticism, but we also have circuitry for kindness, wisdom and courage.

Sophia was also feeling alone and ashamed. She felt unable to share these feelings with Matt because he was so besotted by little Mia that Sophia felt sure he would find it incomprehensible that she too was not thrilled to have become a parent.

With all the glossy magazine images of happy families and beaming parents, it's hardly surprising that young parents struggle to acknowledge feelings of ambivalence or self-doubt. Our society simply doesn't approve of or make room for them. Instead, like all tough emotions, these feelings tend to get pushed aside, in the hope that perhaps one day they might quietly leave by the back door.

Reminding ourselves that emotions arise when specific circuitry gets switched allows us to trust that it's worth working bravely with all emotions. Like Sophia, we too might have strong circuitry for self-criticism, but we will also have circuitry for kindness, wisdom and courage. What ends up getting stronger will depend entirely upon what gets most use.

When we want to work with strong and frightening emotions, we must first build steadiness in our minds. Mindfulness offers us a way to find solid ground to stand on; a safe, warm and inviting place from which we can simply observe all the activity that these difficult emotions bring.

As one of the more respected teachers of self-compassion, Professor Gilbert cautions us not to assume that compassion practices are somehow soft or weak or just about being kind. It is in fact courage and wisdom which appear to be the core personal qualities that are strengthened in these practices.

There are many ancient practices that are drawn upon in the training of mindful self-compassion, but the one I find particularly helpful is the use of imagery. Sophia first built confidence in the foundation exercises of soothing rhythm breathing and body scanning; then together we worked on creating an image she could use in a compassion practice.

As Sophia was growing up, her mother was not really present for her four children, as she was often unwell with a form of chronic leukaemia. She spent a lot of time in bed and needed regular hospital admissions, but in her place Sophia's maternal grandmother was a warm and loving person who held the family together.

So in designing a mindfulness practice that would be strengthening, we drew upon an image Sophia had of this special grandmother.

Sophia's compassion practice

Lying down or sitting upright, whatever feels best, bring your attention to the sensations you can feel in your body. Allow ten or fifteen minutes to move slowly and systematically through all of your body, tuning in to what you can feel in your toes, legs, pelvis, abdomen, chest, arms and then finally your head.

Connect to the feelings of your breath, slowly and steadily moving in and out. With each out-breath allow tension to leave your body.

Now, as best you can, see if you can bring to mind a vivid image of your grandmother. It might feel tricky, and the image might come and go. That's perfectly fine — in time it might come more easily.

Allow yourself to see the kind expression on your grandmother's face, her warm and knowing smile. Your grandmother knows you very well, she is not judging you. She knows a lot about life, and suffering. She understands just how difficult it has been for you to manage this huge transition into being a mother, and how hard you have tried.

Now allow yourself to feel not just her love and care, but also her wisdom and courage, the strength that she is giving you as you allow yourself to be guided by her experience in life and her care for you.

For those of you not familiar with mindfulness, this might all sound a bit unusual and fanciful. But what we are really doing here is using a technique to access and then strengthen certain emotions. In mindfulness we build familiarity and knowledge about our areas of vulnerability, but we also build wisdom and courage, strengthening the circuits of the compassion system.

Another, more traditional, teaching in compassion is the Loving Kindness Meditation, in which certain phrases are repeated. The words that are used are not specific; you can adapt them to whatever feels right for you.

Loving Kindness Meditation

May I be safe

May I be well

May I be happy

May I feel at ease

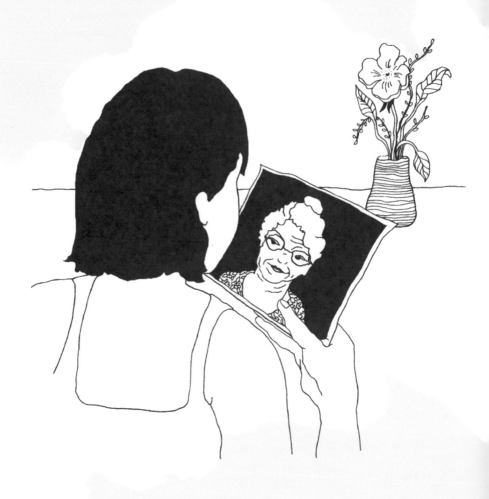

Compassion practice is designed to be strengthening

Traditionally, if it felt comfortable, we would then repeat the phrases using someone else as the recipient—a friend, a stranger or even someone who has caused us pain.

Don't expect these practices to be easy; they can be very tough when for most of our lives we build strength in judging ourselves or striving to improve who we are in some way.

As Sophia patiently worked away with these practices, one of the first things she noticed was a greater sense of confidence with the other women in her mothers' group. I expressed my admiration for her in heading back into a setting where she had felt so alone and judged. However, what Sophia noticed was that as she began to accept herself, she started to relax into being with Mia. When she was with the other mothers she paid more attention to what was being said. Slowly she began to learn about each of them. Two of the women she felt she could trust, and one day over coffee she confided in them a little about what she had been going through, and her initial ambivalence about being a mother. Surprisingly, she did not feel that they judged her; in fact, there seemed to be a new sense of ease and honesty, and the others confided in her about ways that they too were finding life hard.

Sophia was courageous. In her preparedness to face emotions which had overwhelmed and frightened her, she was growing into a wise and humane mother for young Mia.

Reflection

Imagery can be an effective way of activating the circuitry of compassionate emotions. Consider a time that you might have experienced difficult emotions like shame, guilt or fear. If you were to try the same exercise that Sophia used, could you imagine an image you might be able to use in a mindfulness exercise that conveys a spirit of courageous and wise acceptance? This image doesn't have to be of somebody you know, it could be of a spiritual figure or even of a loved pet who is loyal and always pleased to see you. We are aiming simply to activate emotions of compassion, so finding your own way to do this can be very helpful. ■

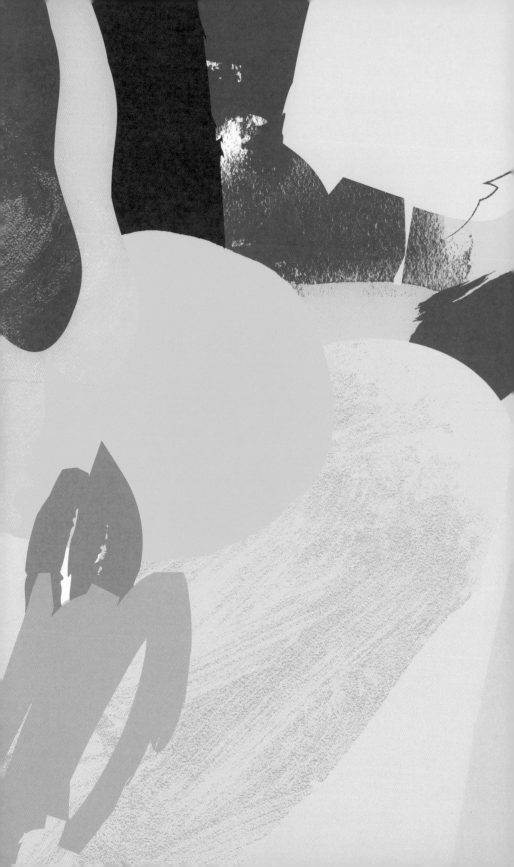

Lesson
23

Savouring and the beginner's mind

> **She smiled and said with an ecstatic air:**
> **'It shines like a little diamond',**
> **'What does?'**
> **'This moment. It is round, it hangs**
> **in empty space like a little diamond;**
> **I am eternal.'**

— Jean-Paul Sartre, The Age of Reason

Imagine this is to be the last day of life as you know it. There is nothing to fear around the corner, you are not going to be separated from anyone you care about. The only thing you do know is that life will never be the same again. What might feel precious to you? What experiences would you want to take in deeply, savouring every detail,

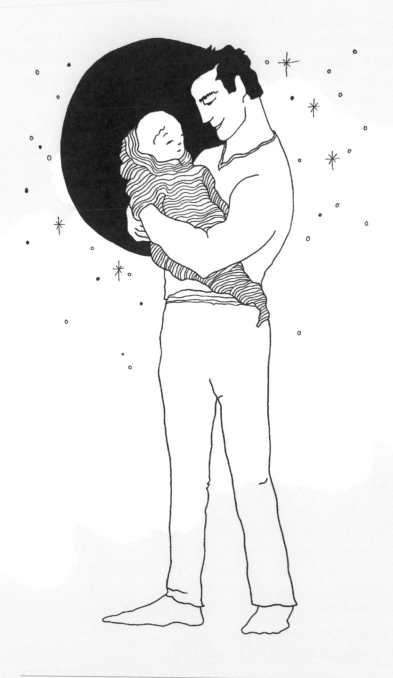

The 'beginner's mind' looks at the world with wonder and curiosity

paying attention as you had never done before? To pay attention in this way is known in mindfulness training as 'beginner's mind'. It is the mind that is full of wonder and curiosity.

It is also the mind that is capable of quietly being with experiences that feel confusing or hard, without needing to race to find a way out or a solution.

Most experiences are lost to us, never reaching conscious awareness. They are filtered out, discarded before they are even registered, when we get caught up in our heads, toiling away in automatic pilot mode. 'Nothing special about this,' a more primitive part of our brain decides, and ensnared by the pull of thinking, we lose touch. The possibility of being intrigued by this moment of our life is gone without us even realising it.

Sean's story

Sean was on indefinite sick leave from his position as captain of a national football team. Knee reconstruction surgery had not gone well, and for the first time in fifteen years Sean felt as if his life was stagnating. And there was nothing comfortable about it, nothing at all.

He could scarcely believe how life had changed. Only twelve months ago he had led his team into a grand final match and won. He had respect, he felt proud of what he'd achieved, of who he was. Now everything about his life felt very different.

Sean was disappointed when he was told by his surgeon that he was not allowed to train for at least six months, but he also knew that this was going to be his opportunity to get into life at home and spend more time with his wife Sally and their three-year-old son Benjamin.

But two months later, when Sean was referred to me, he seemed like a person who had lost his way. Nothing had gone to plan, his irritability was erupting unpredictably at home and it felt to Sean as if young Ben didn't really want much to do with him.

In his career as a footballer, Sean had considerable experience with mindfulness. The team had been supported by a sport psychologist who trained the players how to use mindfulness of the breath and yoga to manage the demands and challenges which were an inevitable part of an elite professional sporting life.

When we looked at how Sean had been using mindfulness, it became clear that the emphasis was one of building attention and concentration. When it came to working with emotions, Sean had been using the techniques to help him avoid being distracted by feelings, which might impact on his ability to focus on the game.

Mindfulness practice now felt impossible for Sean to bear. Whenever he tried to turn the focus of his attention inward with the aim of diminishing the hold that irritability had over him, he felt completely unable to manage an inner restlessness.

What Sean had been practising was not really mindfulness meditation at all. The process of building focused attention was being used as a way of avoiding emotion. Perhaps in his time as a footballer, this might have seemed useful. If he had allowed doubt, fear or frustration to emerge, he might not have been able to be really present to what was happening on the football field. Perhaps; but I'm not really convinced. However, it's not uncommon for mindfulness to be taught in this way in corporate settings.

But I believed there was a way that we could take advantage of the wonderful strengths that Sean already had. Transforming his practice, we could draw upon his ability to be steadfast and strong, and dedicate all of his energy to a cause that had great meaning to him. As the team captain, Sean had a tremendous capacity to support his players, to instil hope and inspire them to not give in. Sean could use these strengths to learn how to be with all the emotions which he had found overwhelming. We were then going to build upon this practice to help him learn a new way of being with his family, by learning how to savour many things that he had previously been taking for granted.

We were not going to tackle Sean's difficult emotions head on. They came with compelling negative stories about how he was failing as a husband and a father. Getting caught up in a debate with the powerful barrage of self-criticism had so far failed to do anything except drag Sean deeper into the activity of his mind.

Using imagery and creativity, Sean began a new routine by starting the day with a 30-minute mountain meditation (see Lesson 13).

In the quietness of his home, while the family was still sleeping, Sean brought to mind the image of a towering mountain that he remembered seeing on a trip to New Zealand he had taken with Sally many years earlier. It had been their first significant holiday together and recalling the scene brought to mind a feeling of love and a yearning to again know that feeling of closeness to his wife.

A transformed practice

Standing upright, balanced and strong, and focusing all of his attention on this image, Sean allowed his awareness to connect to sensations in his body.

He allowed himself to recall a sense of the qualities of this mountain. Its strong foundation reaching deep into the earth, its ability to be still and unmoving no matter what the elements brought. As emotions swept through his body, he paid careful attention to the bare sensations, savouring the quality of each one in turn—a tightness in his chest, an ache in his back; each feeling rising and falling, leaving a new sense of stability as it passed.

As thoughts raced around in his head, he patiently directed the focus of his attention again and again to sensations in his body, and the slow, steady movement of his breath as it entered through his nose and travelled deep within him.

Connecting to a strong motivation to be a father and husband he could be proud of, he then brought an image of Sally and Ben to his mind. Uncomfortable emotions and painful thoughts came and went. Again and again he returned to the stability of his body and the image of a mountain.

Ending with a few simple yoga stretches, Sean imagined that he could bring this energy of courage, commitment and love for his family with him through the day.

As the day moved on—as he began his journey of savouring—Sean brought the same focus of attention that he used in his mountain meditation to all that he did. Making breakfast for them all, Sean ate his own meal slowly, taking in all the texture and flavour. He quietly watched as Ben played with his toast, and chatted away. Noticing a feeling of frustration arising as he looked at the mess, Sean steadied his attention and returned his gaze to take in this amazing sight of his young son. Who was this young child—Sean wanted to know more.

Later, helping Ben get dressed, instead of rushing through the task, Sean allowed his son to take his time. There was really no hurry. Watching as Ben chose his clothes and struggled not unhappily with trousers and a shirt, Sean asked, 'Do you want some help, mate?'

'No,' Ben replied.

Yet something had shifted in the feeling of how they were together. Ben could sense his dad's interest, and from time to time lifted his head to make eye contact with Sean.

As we had spoken about the day before, whenever he remembered, Sean connected with each of his senses. Whether he was looking, or listening, tasting or hearing, he allowed himself to linger with the sensations. As he had when he was playing football, Sean found an inner determination that enabled him to experience the routine activities of daily life in a novel way.

Listening to music he remembered to savour it. Instead of letting it simply add to background noise, Sean paid attention to the melody and instruments. When cooking with Sally, he was present to the detail of what they were doing together and the sense of sharing and being with her in a way that he hadn't experienced for a long time.

Reflection

Try getting in touch with the beginner's mind and dare to be alongside whatever shows up. Trust that *being with* emotion and engaging more deeply in even the most mundane of experiences may just reveal another take on what the meaning of life is. ■

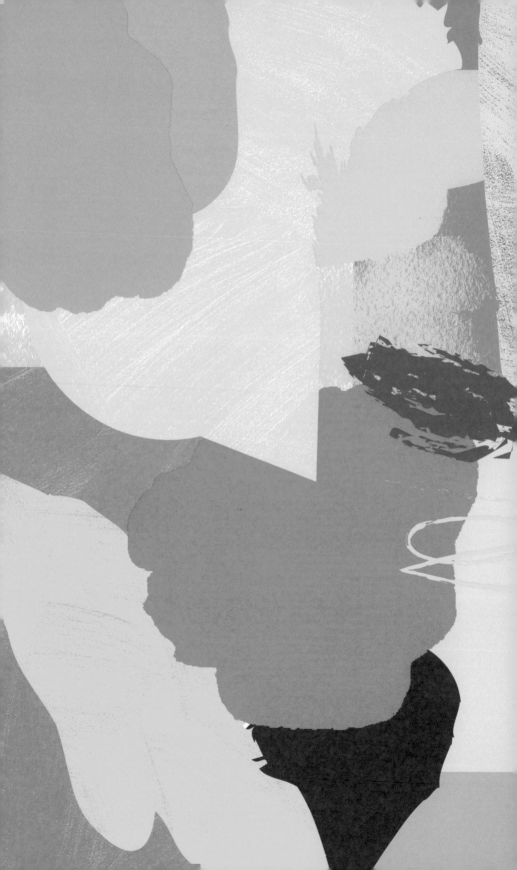

Lesson
24

Attunement

> **"** Your task is not to seek for love,
> but merely to seek and find all
> the barriers within yourself
> that you have built against it. **"**

— *Rumi, Persian poet and theologian*

Wherever we are, whatever we are doing, people around us will be triggering emotional reactivity. As humans, we are all hardwired to connect with others, to want to be understood and to feel loved. The term that is commonly used to describe this process of 'tuning in' to ourselves and others is called 'attunement', and the better we get at it the stronger and more resilient our relationships will be.

In Lesson 3 we looked at research by Dr Ed Tronick, showing that even from a very young age, humans are incredibly sensitive to the emotional tone of their interactions with others. It is in this exquisite sensitivity that the key to building emotionally secure relationships can be found.

Erica's story

When she came back to see me, Erica wanted help with managing the challenging behaviour of her daughter. She had seen me about a year earlier for treatment of depression, and had done really well after participating in a Mindfulness Based Cognitive Therapy course.

However, I wasn't overly surprised when Erica returned with concerns about her approach to parenting, because whenever she had been depressed in the past, irritability in her interactions with others was what troubled her, and those around her, the most. Hardwired into Erica's emotional life was a heightened sensitivity to certain emotions.

Erica was married to Louis, and together they had two young children, Ella who was three years old and Jack who was six. While Erica worked full time, Ella went to crèche and Jack was in grade one at school.

Describing what was going on at home, Erica said: 'Ella is just so cheeky and attention seeking. She's always teasing her brother and nothing I do seems to work. She throws tantrums when it's time to go to crèche and she's always fighting with her brother. I know it's not good, but I just yell.'

Erica was finding it very hard to keep a step ahead of her energetic young daughter. There seemed to me to be no doubt that after finishing her course in mindfulness, Erica was much more emotionally resilient. The activity of her mind was less distracted and the ability to notice and let go of repetitive and unhelpful thoughts was coming more naturally to her. But as many people find, it was in her relationships with others that reactivity still caused her problems.

The strong 'storylines' Erica had were not helping her; they simply added fuel to her automatic reactions. Her view of Ella as cheeky and attention seeking suggested that even if she wasn't aware of it, Erica was assuming that her daughter's behaviour was somehow deliberately chosen.

If it was possible to observe how Erica's brain was operating when she started to feel frustrated or angry and these stories about Ella were triggered, it's likely we'd find strong activity within her threat system and increased levels of the stress hormone cortisol. When that emotional system dominated information processing within her brain, Erica was not likely to be able to think either wisely or creatively. But what made the situation even more challenging was the activity of mirror neurones. When Erica arrived home after work irritable and impatient, everyone in the family could feel those emotions, triggering strong and automatic reactions within them too.

Emotions are neither right nor wrong ... the more we learn to accept them for what they are, recognise and understand them, the less likely it will be that they will automatically drive our thoughts and behaviour.

The situation was a perfect opportunity to build on Erica's mindfulness practice, by teaching her ways to 'tune in' to and regulate her own emotions in the first instance. If we could find a way to help her with this, it would be more likely that she would be able to bring a different sort of emotional energy into the home in the evenings. Then, rather than turning to me for parenting advice, Erica would be able to draw upon her own understanding of Ella for guidance. An important first step though was to help Erica accept that the emotions she and Ella were feeling were valid—emotions are neither right nor wrong.

They may be helpful or unhelpful but the more we learn to accept them for what they are, recognise and understand them, the less likely it will be that they will automatically drive our thoughts and behaviour.

ATTUNEMENT

Erica learns how to 'be with' emotions

Erica chose a couple of times in the day when she would deliberately step out of automatic pilot and 'check in' to see how she was feeling, then put a label to any emotions that she noticed.

First thing in the morning before getting out of bed, Erica noticed that she was already thinking ahead, identifying issues she wanted to focus on at work. Dropping in to the sensations in her body, she became aware of tension in her face and shoulders, and recognised that her breathing pattern was shallow and irregular. The labels she found for this were 'tense', 'worried', 'weary'. If she did nothing more but simply took these emotions with her into the routine of getting the children off to crèche and school, Erica saw how impatience inevitably crept into how she handled them.

On her commute home from work, Erica became aware of how issues from the day were still playing over and over in her mind. Turning her attention inward, she again noticed shallow, irregular breathing, tightness in her shoulders and a vague pressure in her chest. She decided to label this 'anxious' and 'stressed'. Observing herself more closely she saw how when she picked Ella up from crèche, she tended to give her daughter only a brief hug, because she was more focused on getting a handover from the carer and heading off home.

As Erica worked more strategically with her mindfulness, whenever she noticed that she was distracted or her mood was tense, she practised moving straight into a couple of minutes of soothing rhythm breathing (see Lesson 10). Noticing her posture, she straightened her back, lifted her head, and brought a gentle smile to her face. Instead of judging herself, she used a quiet and kind inner voice to support herself: 'It's been such a busy day. It's understandable that I feel tired. All I need to do is simply be here, in this moment.'

In time Erica learned how to extend this softening and opening to the present moment, to her interactions with Ella. She learned how helpful it was to regularly tune in to how both of her children appeared to be feeling. Erica came to see quite clearly that if Ella was tired and cranky and she encountered her mother's own irritability, the scene was set for challenging interactions.

Negative emotions such as irritability, anger and frustration are very unpleasant experiences, and it is no different for our children. Even when their behaviour feels provocative or challenging, it can be helpful to remind ourselves that this is precisely when they need our help.

If you remember from the chapter on the development of children's brains (Lesson 17), it is because of the incomplete hardwiring of their brains that children have much greater difficulty riding the waves of negative feelings. This also explains why when children are caught up in strong emotions, attempting to simply control their behaviour without first tending to the emotion is not likely to work well.

If we bring our own impatience or anger to what's happening, the situation is essentially of one amygdala wrestling with another—not a great recipe for either emotional connection or new learning.

I was aware that with Erica's past history of depression, this busy and demanding phase of her life could potentially lead to a recurrence of her illness. However, we could take advantage of this. When we find ways to stabilise ourselves and step back from the powerful flow of negative reactivity, we are presented with a precious opportunity to actively build emotional resilience. For Erica this came in the form of using her skills of mindfulness to heighten her awareness of self-judgement and to get distance from destructive thoughts. In our work together we looked at the way in which her experiences of disconnection with those around her activated a tendency to judge herself harshly. In her meditation practices, Erica paid special attention to these thoughts and feelings, and whenever she noticed them she patiently redirected the focus of her attention to stable, soothing rhythm breathing.

Erica came to understand that in order to build her ability to be more 'attuned' in relationships she needed to be able to deal skilfully with powerful negative emotions that arose within herself. Each time

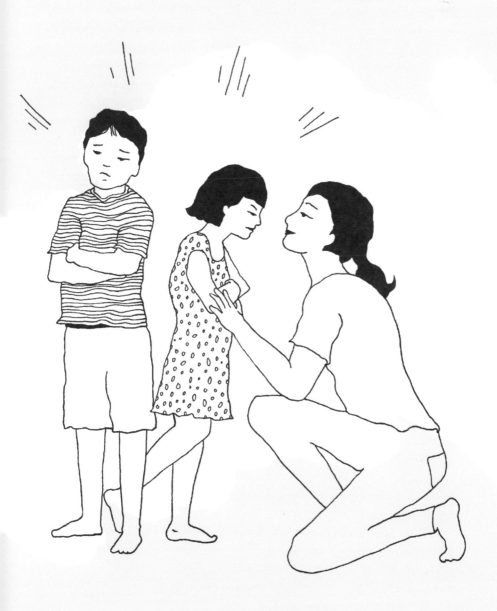

'Tuning in' to a child's feelings helps deal with challenging situations

Erica managed to recognise and not judge her own irritability, anger, shame or fear, and instead be kind and patient with herself, she was strengthening nerve cell circuitry within the connection and compassion system and, at the same time, reducing her vulnerability to depression. Not only this, but the more Erica managed to ride the waves of her own self-judgement and negativity, the more likely it would be that she would be able to help her children do the same. Attunement—the foundation of healthy relationships—requires us to be able to recognise in the moment the emotional experience of ourselves and others.

Over the weeks that followed the beginning of Erica's new practice, she found many ways to deepen her informal practice of mindfulness. She found that even in brief interactions with strangers it was helpful to simply note what was happening emotionally. If someone was warm and friendly, her greater sense of awareness allowed her to enjoy the interaction. If she picked up on irritability or tension, dropping into awareness allowed her to slow down any tendency to be caught up automatically in an unskilful reaction.

Erica found that if she spent even fifteen minutes when she first arrived home to connect with her children and husband, it often made a big difference to how the whole evening went. Having used mindfulness to settle herself, Erica focused on being really present in her initial interactions with everybody. If her husband was tense or preoccupied, she connected with this. She found that catching his eye, asking quietly how he was, then listening carefully to what he had to say seemed to ease his tension.

When she was with her children, Erica came to see that it made a big difference if she softened her voice and her facial expression and made sure that for even a few moments, each of them felt that they had her full attention.

Erica was finding out that family life could be more meaningful and rewarding when she learned how to dive beneath the surface of reactivity.

Reflection

In learning how to build the skills of attunement, it is important to initially turn the focus of attention within, in order to understand a little more deeply what our own reactivity might be bringing to an interaction. In the few moments that it takes to check in with our emotions, an opportunity might arise to bring a less judgemental awareness to what is happening for the other person.

Can you identify a relationship in which you often struggle with a sense of disconnection? Perhaps you might want to plan for the next time you meet with this person, and bring with you a specific intention to be more aware of emotion—your own and what sense you can make of the emotional experience of the person you are with. ■

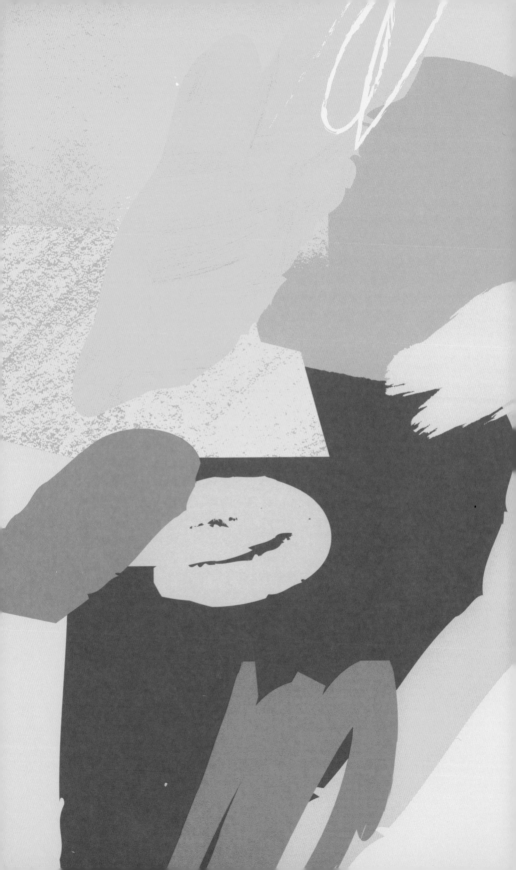

Lesson
25

Mindful communication

> 66 Everything that irritates us about others can lead us to an understanding of ourselves. 99

— Carl Jung, Swiss psychiatrist particularly interested in the influence of the subconscious mind, and a contemporary of Sigmund Freud

When we experience conflict or disconnection in close relationships it can be hard not to assume that something is wrong, that the relationship is somehow flawed. But in reality, relationship challenges are an inevitable part of life, and provide powerful training for more robust connections with others and a deeper understanding of ourselves.

Fiona's story

Fiona was planning how she could get back to her job after having her first child. Liam was eighteen months old, and Fiona's husband Brian was keen for it to happen quickly because they weren't managing to make ends meet on his wage alone. The strain had taken a toll on their relationship, and Fiona came to see me, hoping to find a way to help break a destructive pattern of arguments around whether or not Liam would be looked after by Brian's mother or go to crèche.

Brian's mother Trudy was a vague and highly emotional sort of woman, who enjoyed being with her grandson but seemed totally unaware of what an eighteen-month-old boy was capable of getting up to. Whenever Fiona tried to suggest to her that she thought it might be best for Liam to go to crèche, Trudy would simply dissolve into tears, grab her belongings and head for home.

Fiona was feeling frustrated and annoyed at being left with the burden of dealing with her mother-in-law. 'Whenever I try to bring up the issue with Brian he just shuts me down, and tells me not to exaggerate. I can't believe it. I don't understand why this is happening. He knows what his mother is like.'

It seemed to me that there was probably a great deal more going on than was immediately obvious. After I encouraged Fiona to speak more about what it was like for her to be heading back to work, she admitted that it felt like a very big step. She was clearly worried about how Liam would cope without her during the day, and was feeling guilty that financial pressure meant that she couldn't be at home with him for another year or so.

What added to her worry was her confusion about how to deal with the tension around the issue of child care. For the first time in their relationship, Fiona felt as if Brian was more influenced by what his mother wanted than by what seemed wise for them as a family.

When together we explored what Fiona knew about Brian's family background, it seemed that his mother had always been highly emotional, and had possibly had depression when the children were growing up. After speaking to Brian's sister, Fiona came to the conclusion that the children felt uncomfortable whenever their mother was upset or tearful, and had learned how to do whatever was needed in order to make her feel better.

After Brian and his sister had left school, they both got part-time jobs and left home. Fiona wondered whether that enabled them to get some distance from the complicated relationships they both had with their mother. It made sense then to assume that with the arrival of young Liam, Trudy was enjoying much more contact, not only with her new grandson, but once again with her own son.

If you feel that this is getting complicated, then you're right. Complicated perhaps, but not all that unusual. What was emerging for Brian and Fiona was not at all uncommon in the life of an extended family. As a new nuclear family tries to establish itself, relationships with the new grandparents and aunts and uncles change too. It's as if there is a reshuffling of boundaries all around, and tension and misunderstandings are often inevitable.

No wonder Fiona was feeling lost and confused. Not only was she trying to manage her own painful emotions around the prospect of separating from Liam, but without really being aware of it, she was also being given the responsibility of managing Brian's relationship with his mother. Brian had grown up experiencing his mother's distress as too difficult to deal with. As Fiona was beginning to see, without being able to make sense of his mother's emotional reactions, it was going to be very difficult for him to respond to her demands with kindness and wisdom.

What we have is a family in transition—in fact families are always in transition—because, as humans, we are always changing. However, it is often at times of major change, when there is illness, marriage or, as in this case, the birth of a child, and members of an extended family are called upon to work together more closely, that we are more likely to notice tensions and misunderstandings.

While Fiona might have strong stories in her mind about her marriage, her husband and her mother-in-law, if we were going to be

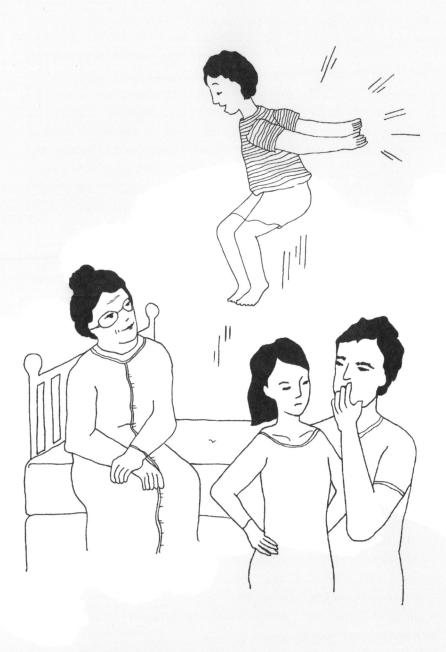

Conflict, though difficult, is a normal part of family life

able to build a healthy and resilient extended family we would need first to address a powerful cycle of negative reactivity.

Emotions are at the very heart of life ... When we learn how to embrace difficult emotions and connect with others from a position of courage, respect and kindness, we are building true intimacy.

It was still a few months before Fiona was returning to work, so I thought that rather than offer any practical suggestions about how to tackle this loaded issue of child care, I would see whether teaching her how to use mindfulness might help Fiona develop a deeper capacity for 'emotional intelligence'.

There seemed to be three main areas that we needed to focus on, and I thought it would be wise to understand and work with them separately. Firstly, we had Fiona's own mixed feelings about returning to work. Then, closely tied up with that, was the difficulty she was having in communicating with Brian in a calm and effective way about the pros and cons of their options for child care. Finally, it was going to be important for everybody that Brian and Fiona together come to a new way of managing the relationship they had with Brian's mother.

As it was, Fiona's tired limbic system was a melting pot of emotion. Sadness, guilt, fear, frustration and anger were the obvious feelings which were all showing up at various times, sometimes predictably, but not always. Fiona had quite good insight into her own sadness about returning to work, but when sadness arose at the same time as frustration and irritability in her interactions with Brian, she invariably ended up in an argument with him, and both were left feeling alone and misunderstood.

If Brian had grown up feeling uncomfortable and at times overwhelmed by his mother's distress, then it was hardly surprising that when Fiona was upset, he would find that hard too. But this meant that at the time Fiona wanted to feel his support, or at the very least have a calm and logical conversation about Liam and child care, it appeared as if her husband was ducking for cover.

In teaching Fiona mindfulness, I suggested that she try to find time each day for a body scan meditation. Building strength in her ability to direct the focus of her awareness away from her thoughts ability to direct the focus of her awareness away from her thoughts and into her body was a good way for her to stabilise her attention, as well as become more familiar with how various emotions really felt. Fiona became aware of a feeling of heat in her face when she felt angry, a tightness in her chest when she was anxious, and a heavy feeling around her heart when she imagined how Liam would cry when she left him in an unfamiliar setting without her.

We used soothing rhythm breathing (Lesson 10) as a practice Fiona could drop into during the day, whenever she remembered, as a quiet way of anchoring her attention even when she was in the middle of a conversation with someone. When she connected with her breath, Fiona also adjusted her posture, softening the expression on her face and reminding herself to pay careful attention to what was going on around her. In this way Fiona was practising 'attunement', or in other words she was tuning in to the emotions of those around her, as well as to her own.

Our next step was to try a different way of engaging Brian in a discussion about child care. It was time for Fiona to begin practising the skills of 'active listening'. Too often in conversations, especially with people we are close to, as soon as the other person begins to talk, assuming we know where they are heading, we get busy preparing our answer instead of really listening.

The conversation then becomes a bit of a competition, as if the best case wins. But long after the issue is forgotten, what usually remains is the feeling of not having been heard.

What Fiona needed to practise was finding ways to help Brian feel more comfortable with making sense of what he really thought about using his mother as a babysitter. But Fiona would be off to a better start if she chose the timing for such a conversation very carefully, which meant not when Trudy had just left, when Liam was often overtired and both Brian and Fiona were feeling tense and weary.

Fiona wanted to make this first conversation with Brian a practice for how they might together speak with Trudy. Rather than launching right into a conversation beginning with her worries, as she was prone to do, Fiona decided she'd try focusing more on positives so Brian didn't immediately feel as if he needed to defend his mother.

Fiona's mindful conversation

On a Saturday morning, after Fiona had put Liam down for his morning sleep, she and Brian sat down for a coffee. Fiona began, 'He's growing up, isn't he? You know, in some ways I'm actually looking forward to getting back to work.'

'That's good,' said Brian.

'Your mum loves him so much; we're lucky that Liam has such a devoted grandmother.'

'Mmm,' Brian said, unsure of where this was heading.

'You know I'm getting better at just letting your mum have her own way of handling Liam. He does get away with more, but maybe that's what grandmothers are for.'

Fiona allowed a pause. She felt a little unsettled with Brian's silence, but knew there was no other way to get to the place where he might be able to be honest about his feelings. Aware that her anxiety was building, she quietly adjusted her posture so she felt more open and confident, and stabilised her attention upon the steady sensations of her breath. Her patience paid off, and it wasn't long before Brian did speak: 'I was watching her with Liam the other day, actually. I came into the lounge room where she and Liam were, and there was Liam on top of the coffee table. Mum was just reading a magazine. She didn't have a clue!'

Again there was silence. Fiona managed to wait until a strong wave of emotion had passed. Then, thinking more clearly, she chose to just say, 'Gee, that's a bit of a worry.'

Brian then seemed to find a new courage to speak. 'I just don't know how to tell her, Fiona. I know you're right. Liam would enjoy crèche and I'd be really worried too if we weren't around when Mum was with Liam. But you know what she's like; she'll take it the wrong way, she'll think we're trying to shut her out.'

Finally Brian had found a way to get in touch with what was really going on for him, and communicate more skilfully with Fiona.

Over the next week, together Brian and Fiona planned how to speak with Trudy. In their planning, they practised how to be with the difficult emotions, so instead of bringing tension to his conversation with his mother, Brian was able to follow Fiona's lead. He spoke quietly and kindly. He paused and listened when she spoke and acknowledged what she had to say. The conversation went better than they anticipated. Even though she was initially upset, Trudy was able to feel his support and affection.

What Fiona and Brian managed to do in their conversations took considerable courage, but this is just as we would expect. Growth rarely happens in the comfort zone.

Mindfulness teaches us the wisdom of opening up to feelings, and making our peace with them. Emotions are at the very heart of life. We can't really feel the wonderful joy and happiness that we yearn for, without also being prepared to sit quietly with pain, anger and fear. When we learn how to embrace difficult emotions and connect with others from a position of courage, respect and kindness, we are building true intimacy.

Reflection

Self-awareness is a wise place to start if we want to change patterns of communication. It's also very helpful to get in the habit of reflecting upon disagreements, not in a way that drags us directly back into the topic of conversation, but more to look at tone of voice, and the way things are said. These styles of communicating that we use can often be quite different from one relationship to another.

Have you noticed any relationships in which disagreement or a differing opinion leads to you becoming more quiet or withdrawn? Is there another relationship where you readily experience frustration and try to more assertively get your point across? Try not to judge yourself. Perhaps experiment with a kind inner voice of reflection, simply describing what you notice— 'I can see that for some reason I felt I couldn't express myself in that conversation.' ■

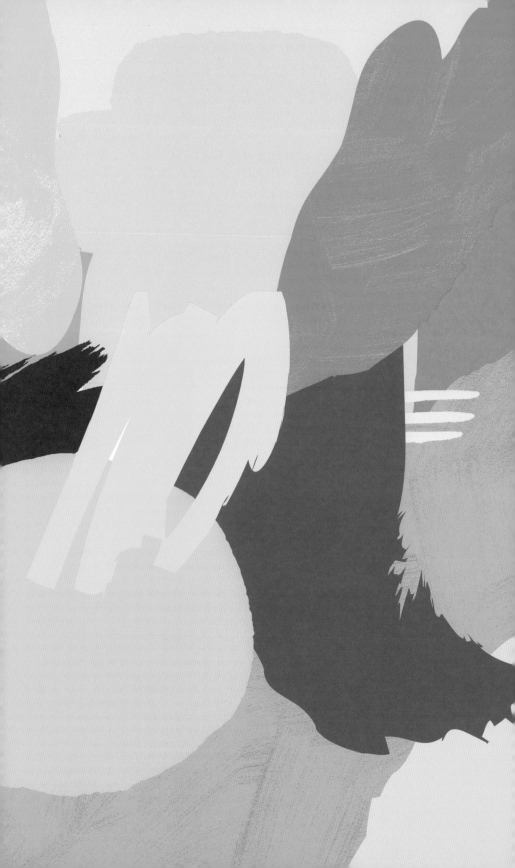

Lesson
26

Mindfulness for two — a PAUSE practice

We all yearn for stability and predictability in our relationships, but in reality everything in our environment, our bodies and our minds is constantly changing. Any desire to feel in control will inevitably be challenged. In fact, the hardwiring of our nervous system is such that as soon as it is detected, change is registered by the stress system as a potential threat. This process occurs automatically and well beneath our conscious awareness, and is the reason why we are so prone to react to change in ways that are not always predictable or in our best interests.

Charlotte's story

Charlotte first came to see me when she was struggling to cope six months after the birth of her first child Ava. Her mood was irritable and the relationship with her husband Wayne felt awkward and distant. In between nightly feeds, her thoughts raced and long after Ava had returned to sleep Charlotte often found herself lying awake, thinking and worrying. She was becoming exhausted.

As Charlotte's sleep deprivation and level of stress escalated she became increasingly tense and sensed that both Ava and Wayne were picking up on her mood. Ava was becoming more difficult to settle and seemed reluctant to go down for daytime sleeps, and sensing Charlotte's irritability Wayne appeared to be more withdrawn and less affectionate.

As she told her story, it seemed clear to me that in the context of her exhaustion and the demands of adapting to becoming a mother, Charlotte was no longer in touch with a more intuitive understanding of how to respond to and connect with those around her. In describing her inner life, Charlotte spoke of a constant activity within her mind, of being flooded with memories of how life had been prior to becoming a mother, and of worries about what it might mean that she was no longer looking forward to the company of her husband.

In the first two weeks of working with Charlotte, our priority was to restore her capacity for focused attention and concentration and to improve her ability to recognise when she was caught up in a cycle of worry which was disconnecting her from what was actually going on in the present moment. Charlotte's homework for the first two weeks was to set aside twenty minutes each day for a formal mindfulness practice alternating between a body scan and mindfulness of the breath. I also suggested that on a regular basis throughout the day she took a three-minute breathing space practice.

As an informal practice, I asked Charlotte to do all she could to be very present in any interactions with her daughter or her husband. In practical terms this meant, as best she could, dispensing with multi-tasking at times when she was caring for Ava or talking with Wayne.

In our third week of working together, I introduced Charlotte to a brief structured practice designed to bring together a number of core concepts of mindfulness, which she could use in an integrated way in her interactions with Ava and Wayne. This is called the PAUSE practice.

PAUSE practice

P—Pause

This initial step is one of the most important components of a mindfulness practice. Simply remembering to hesitate before speaking or acting can provide an opportunity to observe more closely what is going on within the body and mind.

A—Awareness

In this second step we turn the focus of our attention with more curiosity to our inner world, by noticing what is actually going on in our thoughts, body sensations and feelings or emotions.

U—Understand

In this step we observe what is happening in the relationship we are in in the moment. This might be a real-life interaction with somebody, but it also might be a memory of a conversation or an imagined interaction which might take place sometime in the future. Is there a sense of connection or disconnection? Does an interaction feel skilful, uncomfortable or even distressing?

S—See

To see more clearly in the context of a PAUSE practice means that we are attempting to understand the meaning of what is going on, not just for ourselves but for the person we are interacting with. Another way of describing this would be that an attempt is being made to bring a deeper insight into what is happening.

E—Ease

In this final step of moving forward, we attempt to bring with us a broader and more attuned awareness but with a sense of ease and calm acceptance.

Charlotte's PAUSE practice

P—Pause

For Charlotte, using the three-minute breathing space practice helped her become more sensitively aware of the times when she was caught up in her head with worrying thoughts.

A—Awareness

After a few days of practising the body scan, Charlotte felt more clearly how her body was tense and recognised how there was often a tight feeling in her chest. It was in this step that Charlotte began to notice a pattern of judging herself and what she was doing. Each day that she strengthened her capacity to simply observe her thoughts, rather than being caught up in an internal dialogue with them, she noticed just how pervasive this experience of negativity was. She felt critical of Wayne and his withdrawal, and noticed that when these thoughts were present she felt quite angry.

U—Understand

When Charlotte was holding or feeding Ava, she began to notice that if she was distracted it seemed as if Ava too was tense, her body seemed restless and she was less interested in feeding. Charlotte also became more aware of what typically happened when Wayne arrived home from work each evening. He would go straight to Ava and pick her up with a big smile on his face. Observing this close and comfortable connection, Charlotte could see more clearly that she felt lonely.

S—See

As Charlotte began to pay more careful attention to the interaction with her daughter, she went through a very difficult stage of being confronted by feelings of guilt and sadness. 'I worry about Ava. I can see more clearly now how my unhappiness is affecting her.' Around the same time, Charlotte also began to be more aware of how easy it was in her state of tiredness and frustration to bring irritability into her relationship with Wayne.

Charlotte had been working diligently with her mindfulness practices and she was learning how it might be possible to simply notice troubling thoughts, but then let them go, returning the focus of her attention to body sensations or her breath. However, it became clear to me that the strength of these very uncomfortable emotions of guilt and sadness might be more helpfully worked through using a technique of self-compassion.

As practice for the following week, I suggested to Charlotte that at the end of each formal meditation, and perhaps also when she was feeding her daughter, she imagine that her mother was beside her. Charlotte's mother was elderly and frail and lived in a nursing home, but she had always been a kind and supportive influence for her children. Although it was not initially very easy, with practice Charlotte learned how to bring an image to her mind of her mother's face with a kind and knowing expression. She imagined that her mother was letting her know that she understood the challenges her daughter was facing, how hard she was trying and how difficult this time was for her.

As we worked on developing this practice for Charlotte, I asked her to connect with sensations in her body at the same time. In doing this, Charlotte was learning how to strengthen and reinforce the physical feelings that were present when she had this experience of feeling loved and supported.

E—Ease

As the weeks passed, gradually Charlotte noticed more spontaneous change. As her irritability subsided she became aware of an experience of contentment and even joy when she watched her husband and daughter together. A renewed sense of love for her husband emerged, and she found herself initiating more physical contact with him, asking for a hug when she felt tired or worried. She learned how to slow herself down if she was feeling irritable, and pay particular attention to the tone of her voice. With Ava she specifically practised smiling and making eye contact, and this too gave her joy as she watched her daughter revel in the connection.

Reflection

It is courageous work to bring curiosity and attention to times when there is a disconnection in our relationship with others. Do any particular relationships come to mind when you consider experimenting with a PAUSE practice for yourself?

Try not to get caught up with the detail of this practice, it is simply a guide and a collection of suggestions. Even focusing on one of the steps can be enough to bring about positive change. Although with Charlotte we approached each of the steps quite separately, with practice you are likely to find the whole experience begins to flow more naturally and intuitively. Learning how to connect more directly with the present moment, finding an anchor for attention and bringing awareness to raw sensations can be enough to bring about a more attuned connection in relationships. ■

Conclusion

I hope that your journey through this book has been a rich and helpful experience. If at first the practices seem confusing or confronting, try to bring patience to the experience and don't underestimate the influence of kindness. In fact, practising kindness can be a surprisingly direct road to happiness, no matter how challenging the journey of parenting might get.

With mindfulness we learn the importance of taking responsibility for ourselves, how we think and what we bring into important relationships. Whatever spark of curiosity or hope led you to pick this book up in the first place, try to nurture this spirit of inquiry and encourage it. Remember, it is often the most challenging experiences in life which illuminate a path ahead, one on which you might be more likely to find a deeper sense of meaning.

Acknowledgments

A deep heartfelt thank you to all the wonderful teachers who have guided me on my own journey of mindfulness, and the colleagues who have provided support and guidance as I have learned how to teach these skills to others.

Resources

Training courses

Mindfulness Based Stress Reduction—MBSR

Regarded as the foundation course in mindfulness, this eight-week program consists of a two-and-a-half-hour class each week, and daily mindfulness homework. It was originally developed by Jon Kabat-Zinn, an emeritus professor of medicine at the University of Massachusetts Medical School, in the late 1970s, to help people who were suffering with chronic pain and medical illnesses for which conventional medicine had little more to offer. The MBSR course has now been taught across the world for over three decades.

Mindfulness Based Cognitive Therapy—MBCT

Like MBSR, MBCT is an eight-week course originally designed to help reduce the risk of relapse into depression, which it has been shown to do very effectively. It is now used successfully in the treatment of many emotional disorders including anxiety, stress and eating disorders. It was designed originally using principles from the MBSR program, so the courses have many similarities, but MBCT focuses more upon teaching specifically how patterns of thinking can lead to stress, increasing the risk of relapse into mental illness.

There is now clear research evidence that learning mindfulness as it is taught in the MBSR and MBCT eight-week programs is associated with measurable changes in brain structure over the eight-week period.

MBSR and MBCT courses are offered in most large cities across the world. You will be able to find on the internet details of the courses in your nearest city.

Mindfulness education

Openground—An Australian-based mindfulness training organisation.

BeMindful.co.uk—A UK-based mindfulness training organisation.

Websites

www.greatergood.berkeley.edu—This site is a rich resource of videos, podcasts and blogs covering mindfulness, positive psychology and other topics associated with emotional resilience.

www.compassionatemind.co.uk—This site was founded by Professor Paul Gilbert. It has educational material intended for the public and for health professionals, as well as practical exercises and links to other resources.

www.compassionatemind.org.au—This website of the Australian Compassionate Mind organisation provides information about the science of compassion and relevant research, as well as links to videos, blogs and other information to assist mental health practitioners.

www.franticworld.com—This website accompanies the book *Mindfulness: A Practical Guide to Finding Peace in a Frantic World*. You will find free guided meditations and other helpful information about mindfulness, creativity and resilience.

www.tarabrach.com—Tara Brach is a psychologist and respected meditation teacher. Her website provides free guided meditations and recorded talks.

www.iampresent.com.au—My own website contains guided meditations and a blog with links to research, videos and information about how to use mindfulness to promote emotional resilience and stronger relationships.

Books

There are many wonderful books available on mindfulness. What follows is not a fully comprehensive list, simply some of my favourites.

Mindfulness

Jon Kabat-Zinn, *Full Catastrophe Living: Using the Wisdom of Your Body and Mind to Face Stress, Pain and Illness*, Dell Publishing, USA and Canada, 1990.

Jon Kabat-Zinn, *Wherever You Go, There You Are: Mindfulness Meditation in Everyday Life*, Hyperion, New York, 2005.

John Teasdale, Mark Williams and Zindel Segal, *The Mindful Way Workbook: An Eight Week Program to Free Yourself From Depression and Emotional Distress*, The Guilford Press, USA, 2014.

Professor Mark Williams and Danny Penman, *Mindfulness: A Practical Guide to Finding Peace in a Frantic World*, Piatkus, Great Britain, 2011.

Mindfulness and parenting

Susan Kaiser Greenland, *The Mindful Child: How to Help Your Kid Manage Stress and Become Happier, Kinder, and More Compassionate*, Free Press, New York, 2010.

Dr Daniel Siegel and Dr Tina Payne Bryson, *No-Drama Discipline*, Scribe Publications, Australia, 2014.

Dr Daniel Siegel and Dr Tina Payne Bryson, *The Whole Brain Child*, Bantam Doubleday Dell Publishing Group, New York, 2011.

Positive psychology

Professor Barbara Fredrickson, *Love 2.0: How Our Supreme Emotion Affects Everything We Feel, Think, Do, and Become*, Hudson Street Press, USA, 2013.

Professor Barbara Fredrickson, *Positivity: Groundbreaking Research to Release Your Inner Optimist and Thrive*, Oneworld, London, 2010.

The science of mindfulness and emotion

Professor Richard Davidson and Sharon Begley, *The Emotional Life of Your Brain*, Hodder and Stoughton General Division, London, 2013.

Rick Hanson, *Hardwiring Happiness*, Ebury Publishing (Random House), UK, 2013.

Rick Hanson and Richard Mendius, *Buddha's Brain: The Practical Neuroscience of Happiness, Love and Wisdom*, New Harbinger Publications, California, 2009.

Training skills of compassion and connection

Pema Chödrön, *The Places That Scare You: A Guide to Fearlessness in Difficult Times*, Shambala Publications, Massachusetts, 2001.

Paul Gilbert, *The Compassionate Mind*, Constable, UK, 2009.

Russell Kolts and Thubten Chodron, *An Open-Hearted Life: Transformative Methods for Compassionate Living from a Clinical Psychologist and a Buddhist Nun*, Robinson, UK, 2013.

Mary Welford, *The Compassionate Mind Approach to Building Your Self-Confidence Using Compassion Focused Therapy*, Robinson, UK, 2012.

Index

A

active listening 219
aerobic exercise 104–5
amygdala 17, 18, 113, 147, 150, 151
Angelou, Maya 183
anger 44, 45, 75, 125–7, 174, 208
anxiety 44, 45, 75, 131–2, 163
attention 199
attunement 9, 39, 204–11, 219
autonomic nervous system 75

B

beach meditation 134–5
beginner's mind 196–201
body-based meditation practices
    66–71, 86–7, 100–1
    see also body scan meditation
body scan meditation 67–8,
    86–7, 100
    case studies 87, 164, 175, 182,
    218–19, 225, 227
body sensations 100–5, 171, 173
the brain 35, 37, 146
breath-based meditation practices
    74–81, 86–7, 92–7, 140–2, 225
breathing space practice 77–8
Brown, Brené 130
Buddhism 8, 61, 86

C

change, reaction to 224
children, anger in 146–51, 208
Chödrön, Pema 186
Christianity 61
Circle of Security parenting
    program 148, 150
communication see mindful
    communication
compassion 186–93
concentration 199
conflict 214–21
connections 34–9, 44, 45, 50–4,
    80, 210–11
conscious awareness 16, 28, 37, 68
cortisol 20, 44, 113, 147

D

Davidson, Richard 74, 155
daydreams 84
depression 62, 96, 155, 181, 205
disciplining, of children 146–51
dopamine 45, 104

E

emotional intelligence 148
emotional resilience 156

emotions
 balancing emotions with
  exercise 151
 'being with' emotions 206–8,
  210–11
 categories of 44, 75
 in childhood and adolescence
  51–2, 54, 146–51
 cultivating gratitude 178–83
 defined 100
 emotional connection 34–9,
  44, 45
 experimenting with 37–9
 inviting reactivity in 141–3
 labelling of 39, 165, 207
 negative emotions 208
 observing emotions 70–1
 observing reactivity 108–13,
  124–7, 138–43, 165–6, 176
 practising emotions 124–7, 187
 relation to body sensations 105
 relation to breathing 74
 using mindfulness to work
  with 9
 see also attunement
endorphins 104
equanimity 170–6
exercise 104–5, 110, 151, 176
exposure technique 141–2

F
families, connections in 50–4, 80,
 210–11
fear 163, 174, 193
formal meditation practices 86–7
Fredrikson, Barbara 155–6
frustration 208

G
Gilbert, Paul 43–4, 92, 117, 140,
 187, 190
gratitude 178–83
guilt 193

H
Hanson, Rick 17
happiness 154
heart rate variability 74–5
hedonic treadmill 154

I
imagery, in meditation 117–20,
 142, 156, 175–6, 190–1, 193,
 228
informal meditation practices
 85–8, 210, 225
insight 79
interoception 100
irritability 20–1, 44, 75, 208
 case studies 19–20, 62, 80, 96,
  101, 109–10
isolation 19–20, 188–9

J
Judaism 61
Jung, Carl 214

K
Kabat-Zinn, Jon 10
Kornfield, Jack 84

L
labelling, of thoughts and
 emotions 39, 165, 207

Lamott, Anne 84
limbic system 16–17, 147, 148, 218
Loving Kindness Meditation
191–2

M

meaning-making 162–6
meditation *see* mindfulness
meditation
mind wandering 28–31
mindful communication 214–21
mindful conversations 219–21
mindful stretching 69–70
Mindfulness Based Stress
Reduction 9
mindfulness meditation
benefits of 9, 79
body-based practices 66–71,
86–7, 100–1
breath-based practices 74–81,
86–7, 92–7, 140–2, 225
brief practice 102, 104–5
formal practices 86–7
how it works 30–1, 86
informal practices 85–8, 210,
225
Loving Kindness Meditation
191–2
mindfulness for two 224–9
mountain meditation 117–22,
200–1
observing reactivity 108–13,
124–7, 138–43, 165–6, 176
posture 61
starting a personal practice
60–3

see also imagery, in meditation;
positivity; walking meditations
mindfulness of breath meditation
76, 225
mirror neurones 34
mountain meditation 117–22,
200–1
multi-tasking 29, 225

N

negativity
bias towards 16–17
effect of mind wandering
on 29–30
negative emotions 208
negative thinking 116–17, 171,
176
the stress response 17
using mindfulness to work
with 108–13, 210
neuroplasticity
embedding the process of
mindfulness 62
example of 163–4
how it works 9, 37, 187
positivity and 154
returning to old patterns 53,
125, 148
neurotransmitters 44

O

optimism 154–9

P

parasympathetic nervous
system 75
PAUSE practice 225–9

personal interactions 204–5
Peteron, Chris 179
pleasure-seeking 154
positivity 154–9, 178, 179–83
postnatal psychosis 21–4
posture 61
prefrontal cortex 18
pregnancy, emotional stress
   during 17, 19

R

reactivity 108–13, 124–7, 138–43,
   165–6, 170, 176, 205
Rilke, Maria 8
Rumi 204
rumination 116

S

Sartre, Jean-Paul 196
savouring, of life 196–201
Science (journal) 29
self-compassion 187–90, 228
self-criticism 186–9, 199, 210
self-doubt 189
separation 181
shame 189, 193
Siegel, Dan 150, 151
sleep deprivation 20, 22, 24, 62,
   109, 225
soothing rhythm breathing
   practice 93–7, 219
'still face experiment' 34–5
STOP practice 77–8
stress response 17, 42–4, 75,
   86, 113
stretching 69–70
striving 44–5, 75

sympathetic nervous system 75

T

teachers 62
terrorist attacks, reactions to 156
the 'thinking mind' 116
threat-based emotions 44–5,
   53, 75
Tronick, Ed 34, 204
Twain, Mark 173

U

University of Quebec 74

W

walking meditations 100, 134–5
Wherever You Go, There You Are
   (Kabat-Zinn) 10
wonder 198
work, returning to 215–18
worry 174

Y

yoga 74, 171, 173

Published in 2017 by Murdoch Books, an imprint of Allen & Unwin

Murdoch Books Australia
83 Alexander Street
Crows Nest NSW 2065
Phone: +61 (0)2 8425 0100
Fax: +61 (0)2 9906 2218
murdochbooks.com.au
info@murdochbooks.com.au

Murdoch Books UK
Ormond House
26–27 Boswell Street
London WC1N 3JZ
Phone: +44 (0) 20 8785 5995
murdochbooks.co.uk
info@murdochbooks.co.uk

For Corporate Orders & Custom Publishing, contact our Business Development Team at
salesenquiries@murdochbooks.com.au.

Publisher: Jane Morrow
Editorial Manager: Katie Bosher
Design Manager: Megan Pigott
Designer and illustrator: Emily O'Neill
Project Editor: Meaghan Amor
Production Manager: Rachel Walsh

While the author is a licensed medical practitioner with years of experience, the advice in
this book is not intended to be a substitute for personalised, professional care. If you, or a
loved one, are struggling with anxiety and/or depression, your GP should be the first port
of call. There are also great support services and information available on websites such as
www.beyondblue.com.au (Australia), www.nhs.uk and www.mind.org.uk (UK). The author
and publisher claim no responsibility to any person or entity for any liability, loss or damage
caused or alleged to be caused directly or indirectly as a result of the use, application or
interpretation of the material in this book.

Every reasonable effort has been made to trace the owners of copyright materials in this
book, but in some instances this has proven impossible. The author(s) and publisher will
be glad to receive information leading to more complete acknowledgements in subsequent
printings of the book and in the meantime extend their apologies for any omissions.

A cataloguing-in-publication entry is available from the catalogue of the National Library
of Australia at nla.gov.au.

ISBN 978 1 74336 906 7 Australia
ISBN 978 1 74336 914 2 UK

A catalogue record for this book is available from the British Library.

Colour reproduction by Splitting Image Colour Studio Pty Ltd, Clayton, Victoria
Printed by Hang Tai Printing Company Limited, China